Overcoming Distressing Voices

Mark Hayward
Clara Strauss
David Kingdon

16
EasyRead Large

RHYW

Copyright Page from the Original Book

Constable & Robinson Ltd
55–56 Russell Square
London WC1B 4HP
www.constablerobinson.com

First published in the UK by Robinson,
an imprint of Constable & Robinson Ltd, 2012

A copy of the British Library Cataloguing in Publication data is available from the British Library

Important Note
This book is not intended as a substitute for medical advice or treatment. Any person with a condition requiring medical attention should consult a qualified medical practitioner or suitable therapist.

ISBN: 978-1-78033-084-6 (paperback)
ISBN: 978-1-78033-549-0 (ebook)

Printed and bound in the UK

1 3 5 7 9 10 8 6 4 2

TABLE OF CONTENTS

Mark Hayward is the Director of Research at Sussex Partnership NHS Foundation Trust, and a Visiting Senior Lecturer at the University of Sussex. Mark has been working with and learning from people who hear distressing voices for the past fifteen years.

Clara Strauss is a clinical psychologist and member of the clinical psychology training programme at the University of Surrey. Clara has worked for several years with people distressed by hearing voices. She is particularly interested in finding out more about the experience of hearing voices, and is pursuing this work through research and in evaluating new forms of therapy. Clara is part of a research team, along with Mark, David and others, who are evaluating a new form of group-based Cognitive Behaviour Therapy for people distressed by hearing voices.

David Kingdon is a community psychiatrist working in Southampton. He holds the Chair in Mental Health Care Delivery at the University of Southampton. David has published many papers, book chapters and books about cognitive therapy of severe mental illness and mental health service development over the past several decades.

'This book is written in easy-to-understand language and provides a very useful source of information about voice-hearing experiences and how to cope with them. The book provides clear and practical advice about overcoming unpleasant voice-hearing experiences and uses case examples all the way through to highlight key issues and illustrate the variety and diversity of people's voice-hearing experiences. The key points at the end of each chapter really help to summarise the key issues raised.

This will be an invaluable source for voice-hearers, carers and clinicians.'

Professor Gillian Haddock
Head of the Division of Clinical Psychology and Research Group Lead for Clinical and Health Psychology, University of Manchester.

'Building on an established body of cognitive behavioural techniques, as well as the authors' own innovative work on changing relationships with voices, this book offers a way for voice-hearers to begin to cope with their voices and to take an important step towards regaining their lives. It is practical, thoughtful and interactive and will be of help to both voice-hearers and carers.'

Dr Simon McCarthy-Jones,
ARC Centre of Excellence in Cognition and its Disorders, Department of Cognitive Science, Macquarie University.

'At last: a much-needed self-help book for the common experience of hearing a voice. Its sensible and constructive advice will aid understanding and improve self-confidence.'

Prof Daniel Freeman,
Oxford University.

'The experience of hearing voices can be a very strange and frightening one. In this important and informative book, the authors use their many years of clinical and research experience to outline what voices are, how they emerge, the kinds of messages they convey and how we can learn to cope with them. Written in a simple, engaging and very compassionate style, with clear descriptions based on case studies, this book will bring insight and hope to many. Extremely useful to sufferers, their families and therapists alike.'

Professor Paul Gilbert, PhD., FBPsS, OBE,
Derbyshire Healthcare NHS Foundation Trust.

'This self-help book for overcoming distressing voices represents a major step forward in promoting the message that voice-hearing experiences are common and understandable, that you are not alone in hearing distressing voices, and that the key to overcoming experiences lies in developing a balance between acceptance, autonomy and assertiveness.

Links are made between voice-hearing and other common problems in the general population such as anxiety, depression, trauma, loss and substance use. Taking Cognitive Behaviour Therapy as its organising framework and making use of case studies and real-life examples, this guide is grounded in personal experiences. Common unhelpful approaches are described sensitively, enabling the reader to develop both an understanding of why one might adopt these approaches, as well as why they are unhelpful. The authors use "Martin" and "Sarah" as examples, to steer a path through understanding to coping, changing thinking, relationships and self-esteem and finally moving forwards to being the person one wants to be. The important and supportive role of friends, relatives and carers is not forgotten and valuable practical advice and tips are also provided for carers.

A real opportunity is provided for people who hear voices to develop successful coping strategies; greater self-esteem and assertiveness; a more questioning approach to their beliefs; greater equality in their relationships; and in turn to reduce distress and increase independence over their experiences and their lives. Full of practical advice and exercises, based on the most up-to-date approaches, this book will be invaluable for people who hear voices, their friends and relatives, and those working with voice-hearers.'

Dr Kathryn Greenwood,
Psychosis Research Group Lead,
University of Sussex and Clinical Psychologist

in the Early Intervention in Psychosis Service (Sussex Partnership NHS Foundation Trust).

'Hearing voices is a fairly common experience – it is not a sign of "madness" and for many people it never becomes problematic. However, for a minority, it can be an intensely distressing experience. This excellent and timely book is aimed primarily at those people whose voices plague them, but will also be of interest to anyone who wants to make sense of the experience of hearing voices. It provides thoughtful and practical help based on CBT principles to enable people to relate differently to their voices, regain a sense of control and reduce the distress they cause. It is written in a warm and engaging style, and will be enormously helpful to both voice-hearers and their friends and families. Importantly, the authors never stigmatise or pathologise the experience of hearing voices; they are careful to view it as a meaningful experience to be considered within the wider context of people's deep-rooted views about themselves and their relationships with others. Overall this book is a most welcome addition to the excellent "Overcoming" series of self-help guides.'

Dr Emmanuelle Peters,
Senior Lecturer in Clinical Psychology and Director of PICuP (Psychological Interventions Clinic for outpatients with Psychosis), South London and Maudsley NHS Foundation Trust.

Acknowledgements

We are grateful to the people who have inspired and informed our understanding of distressing voices and the writing of this book:

Paul Chadwick for his creative ideas

The people who hear distressing voices who have helped us to learn from their experiences

Ruth and Dawn for their helpful comments and suggestions

Miriam, Milly and Joni for their love and support

Zachary, Jude, Sally-Ann and Ruby for being there

Preface

Have you ever heard someone talking to you, but when you turned around no one was there? This is a common experience. For most of us this experience will be fleeting, maybe a little puzzling, but won't cause us any distress. For some of us, we might hear someone talking from this unseen source more often. We may recognize the voice, some of the things that are said may have real personal meaning, and the experience may be comforting and pleasant. For a few of us, we may often hear someone talking from an unseen source, we may recognize the voice as someone from our past who was nasty to us, and the voice may say unpleasant things. This experience is likely to be very distressing. If this is your experience, this book is written for you.

When we hear someone talking and the source of the voice does not seem to be present, this can be referred to as 'hearing voices'. If this experience causes distress, we might describe the experience as hearing 'distressing voices'. Cognitive Behaviour Therapy (CBT) is one way of easing the problems that are caused by distressing voices, and has been very successful in helping many people. This book uses ideas from CBT to help ease the problems that our voices may be causing.

The book is divided into five parts and uses case studies to illustrate the points under discussion. All names in these case studies are fictitious. In Part One we will learn about distressing voices in detail: what they are; what causes them; why only some people get distressed by them. We use ideas from CBT to help us understand how our thinking about our voices can determine how they make us feel. We also consider these voices in a wider context that involves the way we see ourselves and our relationships.

In Parts Two and Three we introduce practical steps that we can take to reduce the distress that our voices cause. Part Two focuses on simple strategies for managing distress and offers ways to prevent ourselves from feeling worse. Part Three focuses more on trying to reduce the distress caused by our voices by changing the way we think about our voices, ourselves and our relationships.

In Part Four we bring together all that we have learnt and begin to make plans for the future. Finally, in Part Five we look at the impact of our distressing voices on our friends and family, who might often want to help but won't always know how to do this. We will offer them some advice and tips.

Throughout the book, we will invite you to think about your distressing voices and complete exercises that will help you to move forward. Give the exercises a go, and already you will be taking steps towards overcoming your distressing voices.

Introduction to Overcoming Distressing Voices

Why a cognitive behavioural approach?

The approach this book takes in attempting to help you overcome your problems with distressing voices is a cognitive-behavioural one. A brief account of the history of this form of intervention might be useful and encouraging. In the 1950s and 1960s a set of therapeutic techniques was developed, collectively termed 'behaviour therapy'. These techniques shared two basic features. First, they aimed to remove symptoms (such as anxiety) by dealing with those symptoms themselves, rather than their deep-seated underlying historical causes (traditionally the focus of psychoanalysis, the approach developed by Sigmund Freud and his associates). Second, they were scientifically based, in the sense that they used techniques derived from what laboratory psychologists were finding out about the mechanisms of learning, and they put these techniques to scientific test. The area where behaviour therapy initially proved to be of most value was in the treatment of anxiety disorders, especially specific phobias (such as extreme fear of animals or heights) and agoraphobia, both notoriously difficult to treat using conventional psychotherapies.

After an initial flush of enthusiasm, discontent with behaviour therapy grew. There were a number of reasons for this, an important one of which was the fact that behaviour therapy did not deal with the internal thoughts which were so obviously central to the distress that many people were experiencing. In particular, behaviour therapy proved inadequate when it came to the treatment of depression. In the late 1960s and early 1970s a treatment for depression was developed called 'cognitive therapy'. The pioneer in this enterprise was an American psychiatrist, Professor Aaron T. Beck. He developed a theory of depression which emphasized the importance of people's depressed styles of thinking, and, on the basis of this theory, he specified a new form of therapy. It would not be an exaggeration to say that Beck's work has changed the nature of psychotherapy, not just for depression but for a range of psychological problems.

The techniques introduced by Beck have been merged with the techniques developed earlier by the behaviour therapists to produce a therapeutic approach which has come to be known as 'cognitive behavioural therapy' (or CBT). This therapy has been subjected to the strictest scientific testing and has been found to be highly successful for a significant proportion of cases of depression. Furthermore, it has now become clear that the specific patterns of disturbed thinking are associated with a wide range of psychological problems, not just depression, and that the CBT treatments which deal with these are highly effective. So, effective cognitive behavioural treatments have been developed for a range of anxiety disorders, such as panic disorder, generalized anxiety disorder, specific phobias, social phobia, obsessive compulsive disorders, and hypochondriasis (health anxiety), as well as for other conditions such as drug addictions, and eating disorders like bulimia nervosa. Indeed, cognitive behavioural techniques have been found to have an application beyond the narrow categories of psychological disorders. They have been applied effectively, for example, to helping people with weight problems, couples with marital difficulties, as well as those who wish to give up smoking or deal with drinking problems. They have also been successfully applied to dealing with low self-esteem. Recently they have been successfully applied to problem of distressing voices. This book describes the nature of these voices and the contexts in which they arise, the connection between this problem and both self-esteem and wider social relationships; and, most notably, how to cope with distressing voices and, ultimately, overcome them.

The starting-point for CBT is the realization that the way we think, feel and behave are all intimately linked, and changing the way we think about ourselves, our experiences, and the world around us changes the way we feel and what we are able to do. So, for example, by helping a depressed person identify and challenge their automatic depressive thoughts, a route out of the cycle of depressive thoughts and feelings can be found. Similarly, habitual responses are driven by a complex set of thoughts and feelings, and CBT, as you will discover from this book, by providing a means for the behaviour, thoughts and feelings to be brought under control, enables these responses to be undermined and a different kind of life to be possible.

Although effective CBT treatments have been developed for a wide range of disorders and problems, these treatments are not currently widely available; and, when people try on their own to help themselves, they often, inadvertently, do things which make matters worse. In recent years the community of cognitive behavioural therapists has responded to this situation. What they have done is to take the principles and techniques of specific cognitive behavioural therapies for particular problems and present them in manuals which people can read and apply themselves. These manuals specify a systematic programme of treatment which the person works through to overcome their difficulties. In this way, cognitive behavioural therapeutic techniques of proven value are being made available on the widest possible basis.

The use of self-help manuals is never going to replace the need for therapists. Many people with emotional and behavioural problems will need the help of a qualified therapist. It is also the case that, despite the widespread success of cognitive behavioural therapy, some people will not respond to it and will need one of the other treatments available. Nevertheless, although research on the use of these self-help manuals is at an early stage, the work done to date indicates that for a great many people such a manual is sufficient for them to overcome their problems without professional help. Sadly, many people suffer on their own for years. Sometimes they feel reluctant to seek help without first making a serious effort to manage on their own. Sometimes they feel too awkward or even ashamed to ask for help. Sometimes appropriate help is not forthcoming despite their efforts to find it. For many of these people the cognitive behavioural self-help manual will provide a lifeline to a better future.

Peter J. Cooper
The University of Reading, 2012

Part One

Understanding Distressing Voices

1

Understanding voices

The best way to start understanding what it is like to hear voices is by listening to people who have heard voices. We present here two examples: David, who had a straight-forward and brief experience that was not distressing, and Ruth, whose experience is complex, long-standing and at times very distressing.

David Kingdon's story

> When I was about sixteen or seventeen, I was sitting comfortably on a Saturday evening watching football on the television, when I suddenly and loudly heard my name 'David' called. It was my mother's voice but she wasn't in the room, although the call very clearly came from close to me, within the room. It was startling, I looked round but she definitely wasn't there. After a moment or two, I settled back to watching the TV and forgot about it. It was a puzzling experience but it didn't happen again and so I thought no more of it until, later in life as a psychiatrist, I began to meet people who told me about their experiences of hearing things when there didn't seem to be anybody around who could have been responsible for what they heard.

Looking back on it, I was probably a bit sleepy, and was going through a bit of a fraught teenage relationship with my mother: and mid to late teens does seem to be a time when voices often begin. All of these things could have made me more likely to have had this experience. But it didn't repeat and didn't have much meaning to me at the time – if it had, perhaps, been associated with a distressing experience, maybe it would have developed further.

Ruth's story

When I was eleven, my mother died after a long fight with cancer. I had nursed her up until her hospital admission and, while I did not recognize this at the time, carried a deep sense of guilt about failing to save her. Most important, in light of what was to follow, I believed I was to blame because I didn't know how to cook properly and had poisoned her. I was unable to communicate with my surviving parent about these fears, which intensified as I took on the role of cooking for the family. Home life became increasingly violent, as I would often burn the food and would be beaten for wasting money or for making not very good dinners, or for serving it late. Whatever I did was wrong and would result in violence towards me. I ran away and put these difficult experiences to the back of my mind as I made a new life for myself travelling with lots of other homeless kids – until I became a parent myself. My new life became increasingly difficult once I tried to settle down in a house. Both my son and I were repeatedly bullied and stigmatized for being 'pikeys' in the small close-knit village we had moved to. My mental health began to suffer, first with panic attacks and later with multiple voice-hearing episodes over a period of about ten years.

My first voice-hearing experiences were not that distressing. I thought to start with that the birds could talk to me, as there was an aviary next door and I became more and more caught up in listening to them. This was followed by hearing the cats and dogs in the area. I grew up in the countryside and am very tuned in to animals and usually get along with them. Most of these early voices were friendly. But some were mean and vicious. I also live near a graveyard and started to experience the voices of the cats and dogs as messengers from the dead. Gradually, this was replaced by the voices of the dead direct, who I also believed were underneath my house. Again, not all of this was distressing, I heard my mother trying to guide me and this was in fact very comforting. However, there were other dead voices who were not on my side and these became increasingly menacing and abusive, invading my body through the soles of my feet, bubbling up under my tongue and interrupting when I tried to speak for myself. Words really cannot express the fear and horror of this experience. My body became a battleground for malevolent voices over which 'I' had little control. They were torturing and relentless, telling me I had to give up my body so they could live in it; that when I ate or did anything to sustain my life, I was torturing the dead and would have to pay for it. I did not totally succumb to the voices and lose my sense of self completely, but I did withdraw deep inside myself, and an onlooker would have been forgiven for thinking I was catatonic. I did intense periods of silent meditation, tuning in to bodily processes such as heartbeat, breath, digestion and circulation and forgetting conceptual processes such as ideas, thoughts and meaning. This helped me counteract the effect of hearing malevolent voices. It took a long time to come back from that, and to develop techniques to assert myself as the author of the voices and to be in control of which ones (of me) are permitted to speak through my body. Ten years on from my last episode, I still suffer from the intense anxiety and anger connected with these experiences, a feeling that is repeated with monotonous regularity. I no longer hear voices but am still quite vulnerable to feelings of distress when I am reminded about these experiences – and I feel that I don't have as much resilience as my clinical colleagues in managing these feelings on a day to day basis. Fortunately, I now have more 'ordinary time' when I am not being

> reminded of my distressing voice-hearing experiences and have learnt to laugh at myself during the worst of it. Even so, managing these 'reminders' is still a delicate negotiation, and can sometimes lead to debilitating moments between being too noise sensitive to leave the house and too scared to stay there.
>
> *Ruth Chandler 2011 – Coordinator of Service User and Carer Involvement in Research and Development and Chair of LEAF (Lived Experience Advisory Forum) at Sussex Partnership NHS Foundation Trust*

The experience of hearing voices can therefore be very different for different people. For David, the experience was fleeting, straightforward and not distressing. For Ruth, the experience lasted a long time, was complex and difficult to understand, and was very distressing. This polarity of experience is a theme that we will return to many times throughout this book.

What do we mean by 'hearing voices'?

So, what are 'voices'? The term is used as a shorthand for describing the experience of hearing someone talking when there doesn't appear to be anybody actually speaking at the place where the sound is coming from. The voice may be coming from somewhere specific such as the corner of a room, or may be heard 'on the air' or through a window or wall (in which case there may be somebody on the other side actually talking) – or it may even be coming from parts of your body that don't normally speak, such as your stomach or joints. It can be a distortion of other sounds – the fridge humming, for example, or your stomach rumbling. They can be voices that the person hearing them either recognizes or not. They can be negative and threatening but they can also be positive, friendly and useful. Voices are often reported by people in spiritualist settings and can be seen as a very positive experience within such communities.

Quite a number of famous people have in recent times described their voice-hearing experiences. The actor Anthony Hopkins has spoken of how he used to hear a voice saying, 'Oh, you think you can do Shakespeare, do you?' Brian Wilson of The Beach Boys, in an interview, discussed hearing voices over an extended period saying, 'I'm going to hurt you, I'm going to kill you.' Charles Dickens described how he would hear the character Mrs Gamp, the nurse he described in *Martin Chuzzlewit,* telling him dirty stories in church. And even Sigmund Freud wrote: 'During the days when I was living alone in a foreign city ... I quite often heard my name suddenly called by an unmistakable and beloved voice...'

There are different types of voices. Most commonly, they can be talking *to* you. They may be telling you positive things, e.g. 'You're a great pop star'; 'I will look after you'. Or they might be saying negative things such as telling you that you're useless or that nobody likes you (sometimes using swear words). They can also be talking about you in the third person, as if a conversation is going on around you, e.g. saying things like 'he's not working hard enough'. The voices can also repeat out loud what you are saying, or can be just a flow of nonsensical conversation.

Some people hear only one voice; others hear two or more. These voices may talk to each other – usually saying things about the person who is hearing them. But the different voices may also say quite different things and provoke very different responses – one voice may be abusive and threatening, and another may be comforting. Sometimes people hear lots of voices, which seem to be more like a crowd than individual voices.

Voices are not always clearly distinguishable from what we think of as our own thoughts, and sometimes merge into or emerge from them. For example, if we feel negative about ourselves this may be reflected by a voice that is being critical, saying things such as, 'you are stupid' and 'you can't do anything right'. The difference seems to be that you *hear* voices, whereas you imagine thoughts or just acknowledge them flowing through your mind. With voices it often seems that someone is actually next to you and speaking to you – and you are hearing it through your ears. Voices can vary in how loud or quiet they are, and the direction from which the sound comes. Sometimes voices can clearly sound as if coming from outside your head, at other times it may be inside your head or from another part of your body.

Why do some people experience voices but not others? And why do voices sometimes persist while at other times they seem to just go away? Over the past ten years or so, the experience and nature of hearing voices has become much better understood – in large part because we've started to listen to what people who experience them tell us.

How common are voices?

Population studies suggest that many people have heard voices at some point in their lives. Surveys have found that more than 8 per cent of people in the United States admitted having experienced hearing voices when asked the question, 'Have you ever had the experience of hearing things other people could not hear, such as noises or a voice?' In a government community survey in the UK, in which a screening questionnaire asked a question referring to experiences of auditory and visual hallucinations (auditory hallucinations is a psychiatrist's way of saying 'voices', and visual hallucinations is a way of saying 'seeing things'), 4 per cent of the White ethnic group said 'yes' to the question, while 2 per cent of the South Asian group and 10 per cent of the Caribbean group said 'yes'.

It is important to recognize that voice-hearing may be accompanied by other forms of sensory hallucination – for example, visual 'seeing things' and tactile 'feeling things' – and these can be as real to the person experiencing them as voice-hearing. For the purposes of this book, however, the main focus is on voice-hearing, as this is the most common form of sensory hallucination and because working with what the voices say may involve a different approach to working with what we can see or feel.

Most people who hear voices do not have a mental health problem as a result, and never talk to a doctor or psychiatrist about the voices; they may be puzzled by the experience or even enjoy it. But for some people, hearing voices is a disturbing and sometimes very distressing experience, leading many to seek professional help from mental health services. People who don't seek help tend to view voice-hearing as mainly positive and are not alarmed or upset by the voices; they feel more in control of the experience (for instance, David in the example earlier). However, the form of voice-hearing experienced by those who seek help from mental health professionals, and those who do not, tends to be similar in many ways (the differences tend to relate to the meaning given to the experience, and the emotional response to the experience).

Voices and mental health conditions

Whilst most people who hear voices do not have a mental health problem, hearing distressing voices is common for people diagnosed with schizophrenia and other forms of psychosis. So what is schizophrenia?

Schizophrenia is a form of mental health problem that affects about 1 in 100 people. You may also have heard the term 'psychosis', which refers to schizophrenia as well as other related conditions. Although there are various reasons for being diagnosed with schizophrenia, one thing that people with the condition have in common is that they often lose contact with reality for significant periods of time. Losing contact with reality is likely to involve a combination of distressing experiences, including hearing the voices of people or spirits that are not physically present, and having unusual beliefs that other people do not share (this is sometimes called 'delusions'). These delusional beliefs are often associated with feeling persecuted and paranoid – for example, believing that other people are following you and want to harm you. Although lots of people hear voices, people diagnosed with schizophrenia who hear voices will usually have other distressing experiences such as paranoid delusions, and find that the voices and delusions have a negative influence on their quality of life over a significant period of time.

Although about 60 per cent of people who have a diagnosis of schizophrenia experience voice-hearing, many do not talk to their psychiatrist or mental health professional about the voices. They may choose to keep quiet for lots of reasons, some of which may be linked to what the voices say. For example, the voices might tell them to keep quiet and make threats to harm them if the silence is broken. Or the things the voices say may be too personal and private to be shared with anyone else. Other reasons for not talking about the voices may relate to concerns about how other people might respond: there may be fears that psychiatrists or mental health professionals might prescribe additional medication or arrange for admission to a psychiatric hospital (whilst medication and/or hospital care can be beneficial for some people, there can sometimes be negative sides to these forms of treatment). Many people keep quiet about their voices for a long time and tell no one about what they are going through – not even the friends and family that are closest to them – for fear of being stigmatized.

These are all good reasons for not telling other people about hearing voices. However, in recent years there has been a change in the way mental health professionals understand the experience. Mental health professionals working in the UK are now much more likely than a few years ago to know that hearing voices is not itself a problem, that it is only a problem if it causes distress or has a negative influence on quality of life. They are also more likely these days to involve the person who is hearing voices in making decisions about their care, rather than imposing treatment on them. So if you or someone you know is distressed by hearing voices, or if voices are having a negative influence on your quality of life, it might be worth talking to a GP or to a mental health professional.

Why do voices occur?

There are many reasons as to why people hear voices. They can occur when we are feeling sleepy, especially when we are just dropping off or waking up. Hearing voices has often been linked to dreams, to the extent that it is sometimes referred to as 'dreaming awake'. Sometimes when someone you are close to goes away or dies, you can start to hear their voice – usually just briefly but this can become more insistent. Voices can also be heard when people are sleep deprived: experiments with medical students who were kept awake for excessive hours led to many of them becoming confused, paranoid and experiencing voices. Sensory deprivation can do the same thing; for instance, people who went into flotation tanks (which are completely dark and minimize any sort of physical stimulation), would quite quickly – within a few hours – start to hear voices. Hostages are also known to often experience voices. Brian Keenan, the writer who was kidnapped and held hostage in Beirut for four and a half years, described his experience in an interview for the BBC:

> I heard voices – I didn't hear them coming into my ear from outside. They were in the room, *they were in me,* they were coming from me but they were audible to no one else but me. That was scary for a while, then it was very interesting.

Trauma and voices

In general terms, when someone has been bullied or traumatized sometimes the memory of what has been said, especially threats or abuse, can be re-experienced again and again as the voice of the bully or abuser. It is clear that trauma in childhood – whether physical, sexual or emotional – can make someone be more likely to start to hear voices. Distressing voices are frequently associated with traumatic events, with perhaps as many as 70 per cent of mental health service-users who hear voices reporting a past history of trauma. As might be expected, the more traumatic the experiences and the more frequently they occurred, the more likely the person is to hear voices. The voices may start at the time of the trauma or develop later, sometimes brought on by an event such as being attacked – verbally or physically – or by a specific reminder, e.g. meeting someone from the past. Hearing voices can even be brought on by positive events, such as the start of a new relationship.

Drugs and voices

Another common way that voices can start, and then continue, is by using drugs such as speed, cocaine and ecstasy – and, recently, marijuana has been added to the list. These drugs can cause experiences such as paranoia (believing that people are against you) and hearing voices. The effects usually disappear once the drugs leave your system but sometimes they can persist, especially if you experience particular stress while under the influence of drugs, e.g. you are the victim of violence. So voices develop not always as the result of traumatic events – sometimes they can start after taking stimulants such as amphetamines or hallucinogenic drugs. Hearing voices can even be considered a 'normal' experience when under the influence of these drugs. However, for some people the experience of hearing voices continues even after the drugs have worn off and it can then become a confusing, frightening and distressing experience, particularly if they persist for weeks, months or even years.

Voices as inner speech

There has been a lot of research carried out so that we can better understand auditory hallucinations. From this research it seems that when people experience auditory hallucinations the part of the brain associated with speech (called Broca's area – in the brain's frontal lobe) is active. This suggests that there is a kind of 'inner speech/conversation' going on (i.e. we all talk to ourselves constantly), but this speech can be mistakenly interpreted as coming from an external source beyond our control as we don't seem able to stop it or change what is said. It is worth noting here that it is believed by some scientists that 'thinking' in children originally starts as a kind of internalization of ordinary conversation between parent and child. The conversation the child has with their parent, which may include criticism, praise or a running commentary on what he or she is doing, becomes an internal conversation between the child and him/herself.

The term 'source monitoring' refers to a variety of thinking processes that we use to decide whether an experience originated within ourselves or came from an external source: for example, another person speaking out loud. There is some evidence to suggest that if you are particularly prone to hearing voices then you may not be too good at recognizing that inner speech is coming from yourself, and this will increase the likelihood of concluding that the speech is coming from an external source. The ability to differentiate between speech originating within yourself and an external source – in other words, to accurately monitor the source of the experience – is an important thinking skill. If it breaks down for some reason, this may cause hallucinations, including auditory hallucinations (hearing voices). But such a breakdown can be very understandable: for example, if you have repeatedly been criticized or seriously threatened, such speech could be 'etched' on your memory and be readily repeated or revived when you are stressed – thus it would seem like someone is talking to you rather than that you are listening to your own thoughts.

Voices that issue commands

About 50 per cent of people who hear voices hear commands (these are referred to as 'command hallucinations'), and approximately half of these commanding voices are telling the person to do something harmful: for example, 'go and kill that person', 'cut yourself'. The way that people respond to commanding voices varies, and their responses are likely to be influenced by how powerful they believe the voice to be. If it is thought to be very powerful, then they are more likely to obey the command. But this is not always the case. The person hearing the command is likely to be aware of the serious consequences of harming themselves or other people, and this may motivate them to resist doing what the voice says. If a person does try to resist the commands of the voice, they may do this by appeasing the voice. This will involve doing only part of what the voice commands, and is a form of compromising or 'trading', e.g. making a superficial cut to the arm when the voice is commanding them to slash their wrists.

Perhaps unsurprisingly, commanding voices can be very frightening and distressing to the person experiencing them and to those around them. The commands can be very unpleasant, such as commands to harm yourself or someone else. However, there have been a number of major studies carried out which have found no link between command hallucinations and violent behaviour. This is in contrast to stories often reported in the media of someone who has committed a serious crime 'because I heard voices telling me to do it'. If you hear a voice that is commanding you to harm yourself or other people, try to recognize – if you are able to – that what the voice is saying is something that you don't want to do. This may help you to resist acting on the command and instead to seek help, thereby avoiding serious consequences.

Breaking new ground

One of the most important scientific discoveries that has helped our understanding of the experience of hearing voices occurred in the 1980s in Maastricht, Netherlands. Psychiatrist Marius Romme, and his colleague Sandra Escher, gathered together a group of people who heard voices and asked them about their experiences. Marius was prompted to learn more about voices when one of his patients, a thirty-year-old woman, spoke of how she had heard voices in her head that gave her orders or forbade her to do things. The voices dominated her life completely and she had previously gone into hospital several times. Taking medication did not get rid of the voices, although it did reduce the anxiety provoked by the experience of hearing them. However, she found that the medication she was taking also affected her mental alertness, and so for that reason she would not take medication consistently. The voices isolated her more and more by forbidding her to do things she enjoyed doing.

The woman in Marius's study found help through reading a book written by the American psychologist Julian Jaynes, *The Origin of Consciousness in the Breakdown of the Bicameral Mind.* What she read was enormously reassuring to her: in his book, Jaynes describes how hearing voices was seen as a normal way of making decisions until about 1300BC. After 1300BC, philosophers began to talk about 'consciousness assisting decision-making' rather than 'voices'. During Marius's study, both he and the woman herself felt it might help other people if they shared what they had learnt about voices. Accordingly, they appeared on a popular Dutch television programme and asked that viewers contact the television station and share their experience of hearing voices: 450 viewers did so. Of these 450, 300 reported not being able to cope with the voices but 150 said they were able to handle them. Hearing from this last group was especially important in encouraging Marius to organize a congress specifically for people who heard voices and who wanted to exchange ideas about their experiences: twenty people who were able to explain their experiences in a clear way agreed to tell their experiences to others who were less able. The congress took place in 1987 and was attended by 300 people: the range of experiences described by the attendees, and the many ways they dealt with their voices (successfully or unsuccessfully), has proved of great help to many people then and since.

The stories told by the attendees suggested that there are three different phases in a person's ability to cope with hearing voices:

1. The 'startling phase': this usually comes on suddenly and is generally a frightening and sometimes confusing experience.
2. The 'organization phase': the period during which someone develops ways of communicating and responding to the voices they are hearing.
3. The 'stabilization phase': when a person learns and develops more consistent ways of handling the voices.

Initially there is often a phase of fear, anxiety and a wish to escape; this is followed by a period of learning about the voices, what they mean and how to respond to them. Then comes stability, when the voices are accepted and the person has developed strategies for dealing with them.

One of the most important developments from the work of Marius Romme has been the creation of the

Hearing Voices Network – an international network of self-help support groups. This has led to groups being established in many countries, bringing together people with voice-hearing experiences to support and learn from each other – and teach professionals about their experiences. Contact details for the Hearing Voices Network can be found at the end of this book.

How do people react to voices?

So far in this chapter we have looked at what it is like to hear voices, and some of the theories about why people hear voices. Let's now look at common reactions to hearing voices and why different people can have very different reactions. We can separate our reactions into two categories: our *emotional response* and how we *behave* in reaction to voices.

Common feelings in response to voices

People can experience a wide range of feelings in reaction to hearing voices, both positive and negative. Some people feel comforted by the voices while others feel depressed or frightened. For many people, their feelings may change from day to day. Let's look at the experiences of two people, Martin and Sarah, who each hear their voice saying the same thing, but react in very different ways.

Martin's story

Martin is forty-four and lives on his own in a flat in London. He grew up with his parents and older sister and remembers seeing his parents constantly arguing, and on one occasion seeing his father hit his mother in front of him. When he was five, his father left the family home and he didn't see him again. Martin's mother remarried a couple of years later but, unfortunately, this was also an abusive relationship, with his mother frequently being beaten. As Martin became older he would try to protect his mother but this would only result in him being beaten as well. His mother ended the relationship when Martin was eleven, and he continued to live with her until he was sixteen, when he left home to join the army. Unfortunately, Martin was bullied while in the army and, when he was eighteen, he started to hear voices for the first time and was medically discharged.

He heard the voice of his stepfather telling him he was weak, unable to defend himself and that he deserved all he got from the bullies. The voice told him he was no good and worthless and that no one would ever love him. The voice was around every day, although not all the time. When the voice first started Martin felt terrified and stayed indoors as much as possible, avoiding seeing friends and his mother and sister. He believed the voice was his stepfather communicating with him – and he believed that what the voice said about him was true.

Martin has not worked consistently since being discharged from the army. Despite having a series of jobs, his difficulties with the voices have led him to taking time off sick and either leaving jobs of his own accord or being sacked. He lost contact with his childhood friends but sees his mother and sister regularly. He continues to hear the voice of his stepfather, which as well as making derogatory comments also makes threats to harm Martin. Martin still believes everything the voice says and believes that the voice has the power to harm him. Understandably, he feels frightened, has difficulty sleeping and tries to cope by having the TV switched on twenty-four hours a day, as a way of drowning out the voice. In the past he used alcohol to try to cope, but he has not had a drink for seven years.

Here's how Martin describes hearing his voices:

> *The voices are really distressing and they're difficult to cope with some days and I find it difficult to go out when they're really bad. Sometimes I feel really anxious and panicky, and even have panic attacks.*
>
> *When you hear voices it' s very lonely as it's not really something you can talk about to your friends and family, it's something you sort of have to endure on your own really and it's quite often isolating.*

Martin's description is a powerful reminder of the way some people can react to hearing voices. If you have noticed any of these reactions in yourself, it is important to remember that they are very common and that things can get better. Indeed, Martin has gone on to recover and we will follow Martin on his journey of recovery throughout the rest of this book.

Sarah's story

Sarah is thirty-six and lives with her partner and two young children in Cardiff. She grew up with her four siblings and parents, and remembers her family life being warm and loving, if a little chaotic at times. Sarah did well at primary school but started to struggle when she moved on to secondary school. She won a scholarship to a private boarding school, which was some distance away. Sarah began to experience racist bullying from another girl in her year. However, she also had some good friends. She didn't tell anyone about the bullying as she didn't want her parents to worry about her. As time went on, the bullying became more serious, with threats of violence being made – although these were never acted on.

When Sarah was twenty-one she went away to university and settled in well. However, one day while out shopping she saw in the distance the person who had bullied her. She felt a sense of terror and rushed back to her student residence. She couldn't sleep that night and kept thinking about the bullying she had experienced at school. The next day, Sarah was surprised to hear the voice of the bully tormenting and taunting her when no one was around. At first she felt startled, but then dismissed the experience. However, as the weeks went by she heard the voice more and more frequently, making abusive comments but also making threats. She felt confused and didn't know what was happening to her. Sarah decided to confide in her best friend, who was understanding and suggested that the voice was her memory playing tricks on her – and reminded Sarah that the bully was no longer around.

Sarah still hears the voice, fifteen years later, which speaks to her as frequently as it ever did. However, the voice has never carried out its threats to harm her, so the evidence of the last fifteen years has helped Sarah realize that what the voice says is not truthful. Instead, Sarah believes the positive things that her family and friends say about her.

A key difference between Martin and Sarah's experiences concerns what they themselves believe: Martin believes that what his voice tells him is true, whereas Sarah doubts the truthfulness of what her voice says. This difference in beliefs about the truthfulness of voice comments has a huge impact upon the way that Martin and Sarah lead their lives. We will return to this issue of belief later in this chapter. First, let's think more about the different ways that people can respond to voices.

Voices and depression

Feeling depressed is a common reaction to hearing voices. Martin talked about feeling isolated and lonely; he also often felt depressed. When people are depressed they can lose interest in the things they used to enjoy; they notice that they no longer feel pleasure or enjoyment. They may even experience feelings of despair, guilt and shame, or feelings of hopelessness.

People who hear voices might often have feelings of shame or guilt, particularly when the voices make unpleasant comments. This can be the case when the voices remind people of the past, such as being abused or bullied as a child.

Some people who feel depressed notice physical changes such as feeling tired or not having much energy. If you are depressed it is not unusual to have trouble sleeping. Alternatively, some people sleep much more than usual when they are depressed. Some people lose their appetite while others may find that they eat more than usual. Many people also describe having difficulty concentrating: for example, finding it difficult to read a book. If you are experiencing many of these difficulties you may need to seek help from your GP or mental health professional to take steps to manage and improve your mood.

If you have been experiencing five or more of the symptoms outlined below, every day for more than two weeks, then you may be depressed. If you are feeling as though life is not worth living, you should seek professional help immediately from your GP or a mental health practitioner in A&E.

Checklist of symptoms of depression

- *Feeling sad and down most of the time*
- *Not being interested in the things you used to like doing*
- *A distinct increase or decrease in your regular amount of sleep*
- *Feeling tired or low on energy*
- *Feeling guilty or not worthwhile as a person*
- *Poor concentration*
- *Thoughts or plans of wanting to hurt yourself or thinking life is not worth living*

Voices and anxiety

Feeling anxious is another common reaction to hearing voices, as we can see from Martin's story. Martin talked about feeling anxious and having panic attacks in reaction to hearing the voices. When we are feeling anxious we often notice because of changes that manifest in our body. For example, we may notice tension or tightness in our shoulders, stomach or across our chest, or in other parts of our body. We might notice our heart racing, our hands sweating or we may get a headache.

If you are experiencing severe anxiety you might have feelings of fear, panic, paranoia or terror, and physical sensations such as sweating profusely, your heart beating very loudly or quickly ('thumping'), and painful tightness and tension in the muscles in your stomach, chest or shoulders. Many people who hear voices experience feelings of anxiety – trying out the strategies and techniques in this book may well help you to manage these feelings.

Voices and feeling angry

Another common reaction to hearing voices is to feel angry. Although Martin didn't often feel angry towards his voices, there were times when he became frustrated and annoyed and would start shouting at them, telling them to go away. You may feel angry or irritated with the voices you hear ('why are they doing this to me?') or with yourself ('why do I let them get to me so much?'). It is perfectly understandable to feel angry or irritated if you do not want to hear voices or if you think the voices are persecuting you.

Anger can also be a useful emotion. We tend to feel angry when things are not the way we want them to be. So when we feel angry we can identify what we want to change, such as giving the voices less control, and find ways of making this change, maybe by reading this book or by speaking to someone who might be able to help you.

Voices and positive feelings

As we have already seen, some people have positive feelings in response to voices and may feel reassured if they make kind and helpful comments and suggestions. For example, someone who had a positive experience of hearing voices told us how her voices can sometimes offer her guidance: 'When you can't find a way out when you get into a complex situation, they help guide you. You don't have to listen, you don't have to take their advice, but it's nice that they give it anyway.'

We may find that voices keep us company, particularly if we spend a lot of time on our own. However, some of us have positive feelings about our voices even if they make negative comments. This tends to happen when we see ourselves as being in control of our lives, rather than the voices being in control. We will come back to the importance of having a sense of control when we are hearing voices, later on in this chapter and throughout the rest of this book.

Common ways of behaving in response to voices

People who feel anxious, angry or depressed in reaction to hearing voices are likely to struggle to cope with their experiences. There are some common ways in which people experiencing these negative emotions behave in reaction to voices. For example, people often try to cope by avoidance or blocking out the voices, and if this doesn't work they often react by 'getting lost' in the voices (i.e. spending a lot of time talking to and/or arguing with them) and the thoughts and feelings they trigger. We will look at these two common behavioural reactions one by one and then address more helpful ways to respond to voices.

Avoidance

It is understandable that people want to avoid and withdraw from unpleasant experiences. We all do this when we're confronted by a situation that we don't feel able or want to change, e.g. avoiding a friend we have fallen out with. If you are hearing voices and the experience is making you feel depressed, angry or anxious, it is quite likely that you will try to find ways of avoiding the voices. This might involve staying indoors as much as possible, which may have the consequences of stopping you from working, seeing friends and family, or doing other enjoyable activities. We saw earlier that Martin stayed indoors in response to the things the voices said. Staying indoors is a common reaction when we feel depressed, because we lack energy or have feelings of hopelessness. It is also a common reaction when you feel anxious, particularly when you have anxious thoughts about what might happen in the outside world. For example, if the voices say that going outside is dangerous and you will be attacked, bullied or harmed, it may feel natural and sensible to try to protect yourself by staying indoors. However, staying indoors can lead you to feel depressed, not least because you miss out on doing enjoyable, meaningful activities and spend less time with your friends and family. So, in the long term, staying indoors is often not a very helpful strategy.

Another common way of trying to avoid unpleasant experiences is to try and block them out. Some people do this by sleeping as much as possible, by going to bed early and getting up late or perhaps by sleeping during the day. For some, when you're asleep might be the only time when the voices are not around, and so sleeping can seem like an effective way of getting rid of them for a short time. Some people who hear voices say that they stop or become less noticeable when they're watching television or listening to music: thus this can be a helpful way of coping for some people. A downside to coping with voices by sleeping a lot, or by excessively pursuing one activity such as watching television, means that you can miss out on doing the things you really enjoy.

Other ways of blocking out voices include drinking alcohol or using recreational drugs. The downside to this strategy is that drinking alcohol and using drugs can have the undesired effect of making the voices occur more frequently. This can lead to using more alcohol or drugs in order to try to cope with this consequence, and so a vicious cycle develops as the voices become more intense and more alcohol or drugs are used in an effort to cope with them.

Trying to block out or stop the voices is often not very effective and can sometimes make voices come back more intensely and more loudly. A quick and easy experiment to demonstrate this is to try *not* thinking about a white rabbit for a few moments and seeing what happens. Chances are you found yourself thinking about white rabbits! This is a good demonstration of the general rule that when we try to not think about something our minds seem to become more aware of the thing we're trying to avoid and so we think about it even more!

'Getting lost' in the voices

Often, avoiding voices or trying to block them out does not work and people end up 'getting lost' in the voices. What we mean by this is that we may end up spending a lot of time, perhaps hours every day, listening to the voices and maybe talking or arguing with them. As you can imagine, 'getting lost' in the voices stops us from doing enjoyable things in our life that give us a sense of meaning and pleasure, simply because so much time is spent engaging with the voices.

Some people say that arguing with the voices can help them to feel better for a while – as at least they are doing something by standing up to the voices. Other people say that the voices can, in fact, get worse when they argue with them, causing them to feel more depressed, angry or anxious.

As well as getting lost in the voices, people can also get lost in thoughts and feelings. What we mean by this is that we might find we spend a lot of time thinking about why we hear the voices or why our lives are the way they are. We might spend hours caught up in negative thoughts and feelings or worrying about the future. Sometimes these negative thoughts might be aimed directly at ourselves, or they might be thoughts or worries about other people, or more general concerns such as the world being a dangerous and unsafe place. Just as engaging with voices can make us feel more depressed or more anxious, so too can engaging with negative thoughts and feelings. In Parts Two and Three of this book we will explore ways of coping with voices without getting caught up with and lost in these experiences.

Helpful ways of responding to voices

As we have seen, many people who hear voices cope well with their experiences and some people even find that the voices have a positive influence in their lives. Marius Romme and his colleague Sandra Escher found that people who coped well with voices often had good relationships with their families and friends, were still working and had a range of enjoyable hobbies. An important difference between people who coped well and those who did not was in each group's sense of control. People who coped well tended to see themselves as stronger than the voices, whereas those who did not cope so well often said that the voices were stronger than them.

Why do voices cause distress?

As already outlined, for some people hearing voices can be a positive and valued experience that, in some cases, is even encouraged. In such instances, the voices are likely to be engaged with and welcomed. For other people, the voices can be upsetting and cause anxiety or depression. So what leads one person to experience their voices as positive and a source of pleasure, and another to find them distressing?

Broadly speaking, how we react to hearing voices depends on what we believe about the voices and ourselves. Beliefs are not facts, they are best guesses, but they can influence how we think. Some of our beliefs about voices relate to power and control. We might believe that voices are all-powerful ('omnipotent') and can control our feelings and behaviour. For example, it is often believed that voices can make bad things happen or make us behave in certain ways that cause harm to ourselves or others (such as the commanding voices discussed earlier). However, believing that voices have power over us tends to cause most distress if we also believe that the voices intend to harm us ('malevolence') and if we believe that we are powerless against them. If you believe that a voice is powerful but also that it only has positive intentions towards you – to guide and comfort you – then it is unlikely to cause you much distress. Similarly, if you believe that a voice is powerful and intends to harm you but that you are powerful enough to resist it and stay in control, by not obeying its commands, it is likely to cause you less distress than if you believed you were under its control and could not resist its commands. In this sense, what causes problems is not your beliefs about the power of the voices, but rather a combination of your beliefs about the power of the voice, your beliefs about the voice's intentions towards you, and your beliefs about your own power. This is illustrated in Figure 1:

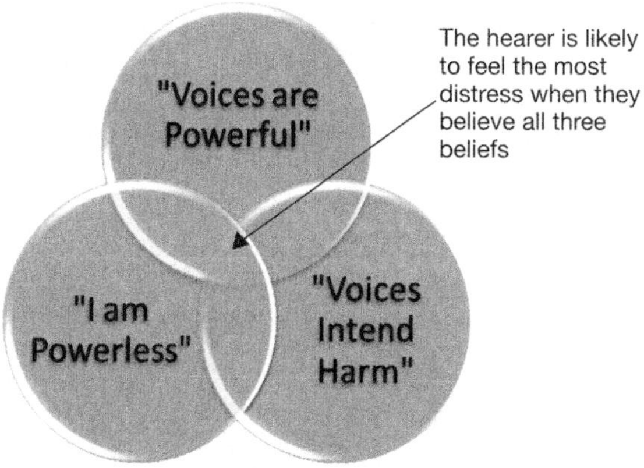

Figure 1: The interaction between beliefs

Another belief that will affect how distressing we find the experience of hearing voices relates to how *truthful* we perceive the voices to be. Many people who hear voices report that they make very negative and personal comments about them. Unsurprisingly, if we believe these comments, we're likely to find them extremely upsetting. If you already have a negative view of yourself – for example, if you consider yourself worthless and unlovable – you're more likely to accept the negative comments of the voices: they may even strengthen your negative views of yourself. The very personal nature of the comments made by voices can be very influential, precisely because they can be *so* personal that they can sometimes be perceived as being all-knowing (omniscient). If the voices seem to know everything, you are more likely to believe that they are very powerful.

Cognitive Behaviour Therapy for hearing voices

The diagram in Figure 2 illustrates the relationship between our experiences, thoughts, feelings and reactions. Understanding this relationship provides the basis for the therapy on which this book is based – Cognitive Behaviour Therapy (CBT). CBT is a form of therapy that helps us to understand our experiences by separating out thoughts, feelings, bodily sensations and behaviour, and seeing how these four aspects of our experience influence each other. According to the CBT approach, if we have negative thoughts we are then likely to have negative feelings, notice unpleasant sensations in our bodies and then behave in ways that might make us feel worse as we try to cope with these difficult experiences.

When someone hears voices (shown as 'A' in the diagram), how they feel and how they behave (shown as 'C' in the diagram) will depend in part on what they believe about the voices (shown as 'B' in the diagram).

You might remember the survey conducted by Marius Romme and Sandra Escher, discussed earlier in this chapter. They found that more than one-third of people who took part in their survey were *not* distressed by hearing voices, while the other two-thirds of people who took part *did* find the experience of hearing voices upsetting. Figure 2 can help us to understand this difference. We have seen that what makes the difference between feeling okay about the voices, or feeling depressed and anxious, is partly to do with what we *believe* about the voices: we know that if people believe that voices have power over them then they are much more likely to feel distressed.

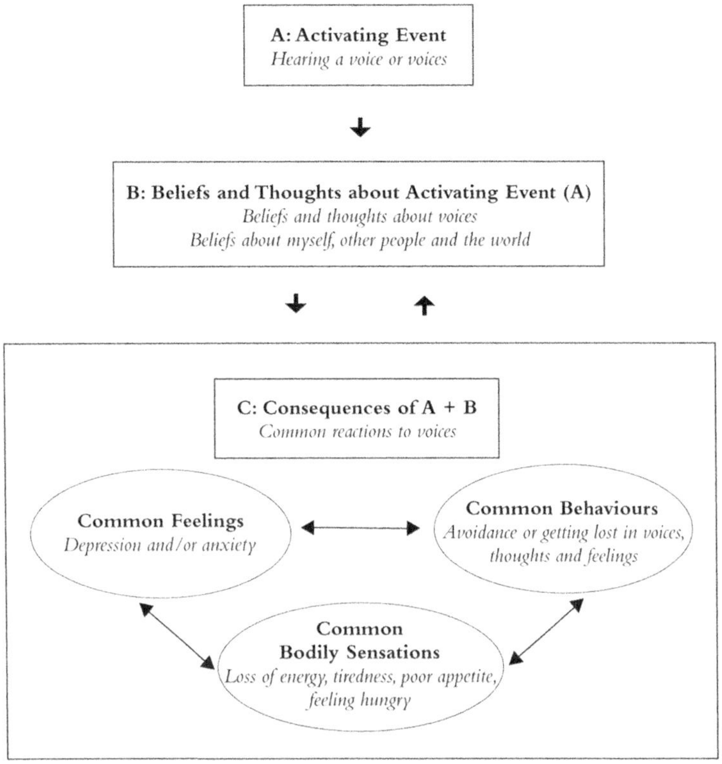

Figure 2: CBT for hearing voices – the ABC model, used with permission, Chadwick, P., Birchwood, M. & Trower, P. Cognitive Therapy for delusions, voices and paranoia. Chichester: Wiley

Let's illustrate this point by applying the ABC model to Martin and Sarah's experiences.

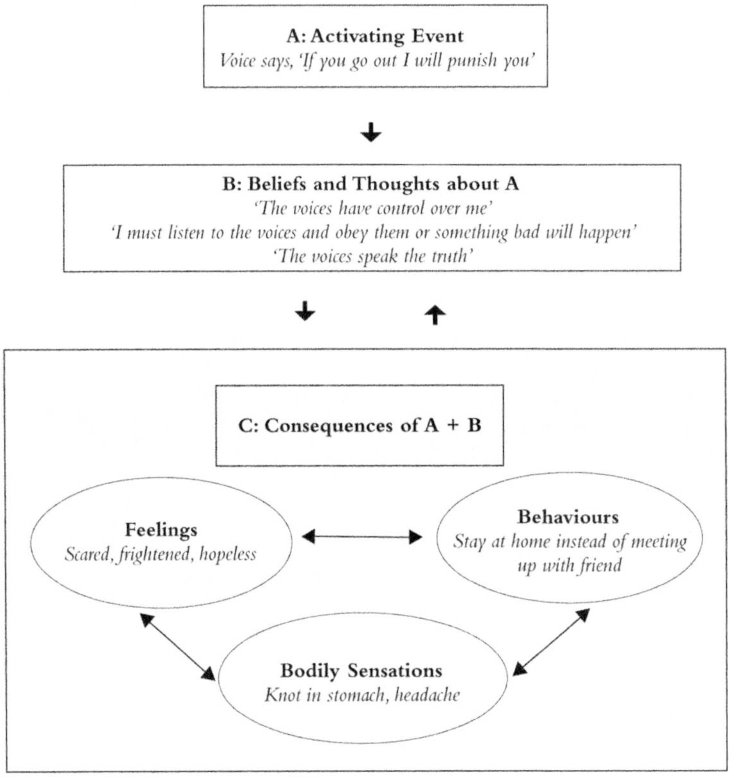

Figure 3: Martin

As we can see in Figure 3 above, Martin believes that the voices have control over him and that he must obey what they say or something bad will happen. It makes sense, therefore, that he feels scared and decides to stay at home rather than meet his friend. In contrast, in Figure 4 we can see that Sarah believes the voices have no control over her and that they cannot make bad things happen. In this case, it makes sense that she feels empowered and proud of herself (if a little irritated by the voices) as she decides to go out, despite what the voice says.

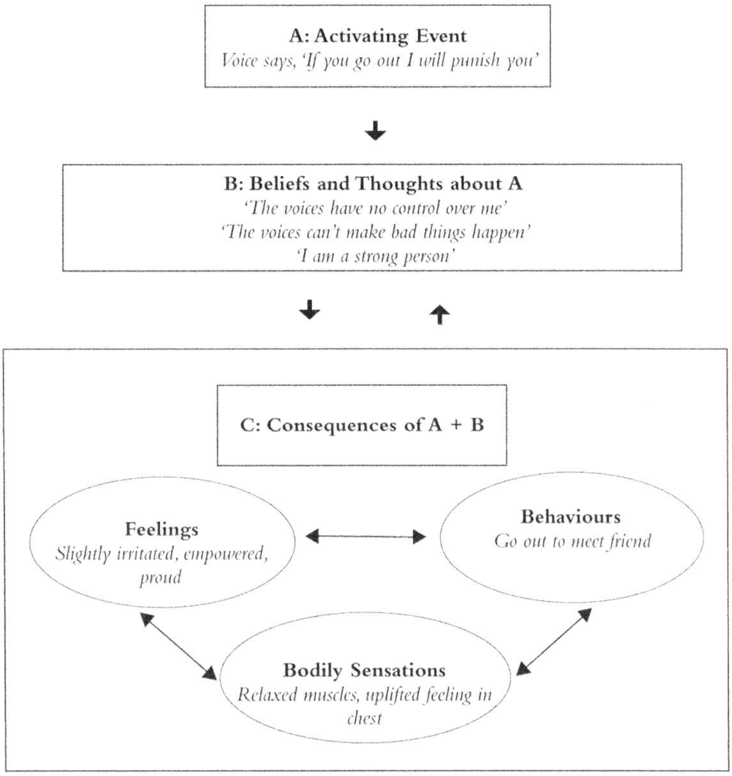

Figure 4: Sarah

We will refer to Martin's experiences throughout Parts 2, 3 and 4 of this book as we try to illustrate many of the different ways of coping with and trying to change voice-hearing experiences. By regularly referring to Martin's experiences we are not suggesting that he (or you) should try every activity suggested in this book. Instead, we hope that you will become familiar with his experience of hearing voices and that this will clearly illustrate many of the techniques and strategies that are described.

What other treatments are available for hearing distressing voices?

Whilst the focus of this book is CBT, there are a range of treatments that are available in order to try to reduce the distress and disturbance to your quality of life that hearing voices may cause. Some of these other treatments are briefly described below.

Medication

There are medications available that can reduce voice activity and which might help to reduce feelings of anxiety or depression. Some people who are distressed by hearing voices seem to find medication a helpful treatment whereas other people find that medication does not make much difference. There are also side effects to most of the medications, which means that some people don't want to take them for a long period of time. If you, or someone you know, are feeling distress because of hearing voices then it would be worth talking to a GP or a mental health professional about what medication options might be available and about the pros and cons of taking medication. The important issue of medication is considered in more detail in Chapter 4.

Support groups

The Hearing Voices Network is an active and thriving organization run by and for people who hear voices, sometimes in conjunction with mental health professionals. Support groups operate in many parts of the UK and around the world (see the list of useful organizations provided at the end of the book for contact details). They are an opportunity to meet other people who hear voices, to talk about the experience and to share ideas about ways of coping with and managing voices. People who go to these groups usually find them very helpful and supportive.

Individual psychological therapy

The ideas in this book are drawn from Cognitive Behaviour Therapy (CBT). This is a form of therapy that can help us to change our behaviour so that we do more of the things we find helpful and fewer of the things that are unhelpful. The therapy also helps us to look at and evaluate our unhelpful thinking patterns and beliefs.

CBT has been used in the treatment of distressing voices, and research has found that this form of therapy can be very helpful for many people in reducing feelings of distress, increasing self-esteem and in improving quality of life. In 2009, the Department of Health in the UK recommended that people with a diagnosis of schizophrenia should be offered at least sixteen individual CBT sessions by the NHS. If you would like to find out about this, either speak to your GP or to a mental health professional.

Family therapy

If someone is hearing distressing voices this is also likely to be a difficult experience for their partner, children, parents and friends. Family therapy can be a very useful opportunity for families to work together to find the best ways of supporting each other. There is plenty of research evidence showing that family therapy for people who hear distressing voices can help to keep people well for longer and can help families to get along better with each other. A GP or a mental health professional will be able to tell you about family therapy that might be available in your local area.

Art therapy

Sometimes when people hear distressing voices they can also feel very tired, lacking in energy and can find it hard to motivate themselves to do the things they used to do. When this happens, art therapy can be helpful. The 2009 Department of Health guidelines recommend that art therapy is offered to people when they have a diagnosis of schizophrenia and when they have an extreme lack of energy or motivation. If you or someone you know would like to find out more about this you may wish to speak to a GP or a mental health professional.

Summary

In this chapter, we have learnt ways to understand voices: what they are, what can cause them, how we think about them and how they make us feel. We have also learnt about ourselves: how we think about ourselves and how this can impact upon the way voices make us feel. In the next chapter, we will begin to look more closely at the way we think about ourselves. If we can understand and change ways of thinking about ourselves, then we will be likely to feel less distressed by what voices say. We will be able to start doing the things we want to do in order to have a meaningful and rewarding life.

Key points

- Voices is a shorthand for describing the experience of hearing someone talking when there doesn't appear to be anybody actually speaking from where the sound is coming.
- Hearing voices is quite common, and has been experienced by many well-known people.
- Voices can occur for many reasons – including traumatic childhood experiences, sleepiness and sensory deprivation, drug use, or problematic thinking and how we process difficult thoughts.

- Many people who hear voices are not upset by them and cope well. Some people even find their voices to be a positive experience.
- When the voices are upsetting, they can cause depression, anxiety and anger. One common reaction is to try to avoid the voices. If this is not successful, we can 'get lost in voices' by listening to them and arguing with them.
- How we respond to the voices we hear can depend on what we believe about the voices and what we believe about ourselves. If we believe voices are all-powerful and intend to harm us – and that we have no control over them – we are likely to be distressed.
- Cognitive Behaviour Therapy (CBT) focuses on understanding and changing beliefs about our voices and ourselves.
- CBT is one of a number of treatments that may help someone who is distressed by hearing voices. It is important to find the treatment that is right for you.

2

Self-esteem and hearing voices

So far we have looked at why some people hear voices when no one is around. We have seen that different people have very different reactions to hearing voices – some people are comforted by voices while others find voices very upsetting. We saw that an important reason for this difference is that some people believe that voices are controlling, powerful and want to cause harm, whereas other people think that voices have good intentions and do not have any real power or control.

In this chapter, we look at the impact of hearing voices on self-esteem. Low self-esteem (which involves having strong negative ideas about who we are) and being distressed by hearing voices usually go hand in hand. In this chapter, we will look at what we mean by low self-esteem, why low self-esteem develops in the first place and what keeps it going. Finally we look at why low self-esteem and feeling distressed by voices often go together.

What is low self-esteem?

Do I have low self-esteem?

We all have ideas and opinions about the kind of person we are. These might be facts about ourselves that we do not feel particularly strongly about, such as 'I have brown hair', or other ideas and opinions about ourselves that carry more emotional weight. Low self-esteem is when our overall view of ourselves is negative. Have a look at the statements in Table 1 in order to form an impression of your own self-esteem. For each statement, you might want to decide whether or not you think it is true for you by ticking the most appropriate box on the right-hand side.

How did you respond to these statements? Add up the scores for each item you ticked: the maximum possible score is 30, which equals the highest level of self-esteem. The lower the score the lower your self-esteem. The average score in the general population is around 22 or 23, although this can vary quite a lot. The majority of people score between 17 and 28[1] on the questionnaire, so if you score less

---

1 Sinclair, S.J., Blais, M.A., Gansler, D.A., Sandberg, E., Bistis, K. & LoCicero, A. (2010). 'Psychometric properties of the Rosenberg Self-Esteem Scale: Overall and across demographic groups living within the United States'. Evaluation & the Health Professions, 33, 56–80.

than 17 this might mean that you have lower self-esteem than most. This is based on data from a paper by Sinclair et al. (2010) who conducted a representative, general population survey in the US.

After looking through the statements and calculating your score you might realize that low self-esteem is not a problem for you. On the other hand, you might realize that you have some problems with low self-esteem and you may find the ideas in this chapter helpful.

Table 1: Rating your self-esteem (Rosenberg Self-Esteem Scale, Rosenberg 1965)

1. On the whole I am satisfied with myself.

Strongly Agree

3

Agree

2

Disagree

1

Strongly disagree

0

2. At times, I think I am no good at all.

Strongly Agree

0

Agree

1

Disagree

2

Strongly disagree

3

3. I feel that I have a number of good qualities.

Strongly Agree

3

Agree

2

Disagree

1

Strongly disagree

0

4. I am able to do things as well as most other people.

Strongly Agree

3

Agree

2

Disagree

1

Strongly disagree

0

5. I feel I do not have much to be proud of.

Strongly Agree

0

Agree

1

Disagree

2

Strongly disagree

3

6. I certainly feel useless at times.

Strongly Agree

0

Agree

1

Disagree

2

Strongly disagree

3

7. I feel that I'm a person of worth, at least on an equal plane with others.

Strongly Agree

3

Agree

2

Disagree

1

Strongly disagree

0

8. I wish I could have more respect for myself.

Strongly Agree

0

Agree

1

Disagree

2

Strongly disagree

3

9. All in all, I am inclined to feel that I am a failure.

Strongly Agree

0

Agree

1

Disagree

2

Strongly disagree

3

10. I take a positive attitude towards myself.

Strongly Agree

3

Agree

2

Disagree

1

Strongly disagree

0

Total score=_____/30

(The higher the score the higher the self-esteem)

Negative core beliefs

Low self-esteem involves having a negative opinion of ourselves. At the heart of this lies negative beliefs about who we are as a person. When negative beliefs seem true – when they make us feel strongly and when they have been around a long time (often since we were young children) – we can call them 'core beliefs'. They are called 'core beliefs' in CBT because they are at the very centre of what we believe about ourselves as a person.[2] Negative core beliefs lie at the very centre of low self-esteem.

Here are some common core beliefs:

- I am kind
- I am no good
- I am clever
- I am stupid

---

2 We can also have core beliefs about other people and the world in general. In this chapter we are focusing on core beliefs about ourselves.

- I am weak
- I am vulnerable
- I am strong
- I am capable
- I am unlovable
- I am worthwhile

From this list, we can see two things. First, that core beliefs about ourselves can be worded as 'I am...' statements, and that these statements say something that seems to be true all of the time (thus the truth of core beliefs does not change from one situation to the next). Second, core beliefs can be positive or negative. In this chapter, we will focus on negative core beliefs. Later on, in Chapter 6, we look more at building up positive core beliefs as a way of overcoming distressing voices.

If you look at the negative core beliefs in the list can you think of someone you know who might believe some of these things about themselves? Do you agree with this person's view of themselves? Often we do not agree with someone's negative view of themselves. So although negative core beliefs about ourselves can seem completely true to us, they usually are not how other people see us.

Do you recognize in yourself any of the negative core beliefs in the list? When you consider these core beliefs how do you feel? Do you believe they are true about you? Do you know anyone who would disagree with you about this negative view of yourself? What would they say to you? These questions highlight that negative core beliefs can seem completely true to us about ourselves, but not at all true to other people in how they think about us. So, if negative core beliefs are not accurate ways of viewing ourselves, then where do they come from and why do they develop in the first place?

Where does low self-esteem come from?

Low self-esteem and life experiences

We have already seen that our negative core beliefs often seem completely true. They seem true for a good reason – and that is because we usually develop core beliefs when we are young children, as a way of making sense of our life experiences.

Have a think for a moment if you know any young children, say aged between two and five years old. If you can't think of any young children you know at the moment, perhaps think of young children you've known in the past. Or you might be able to remember what it was like to be a young child yourself.

What do young children do when a trusted adult tells them something is true? How about when we tell young children about Santa Claus or the Tooth Fairy?

Children tend to believe what people tell them, especially when that person is someone they trust. It makes perfect sense for children to believe what adults tell them, because they have so much to learn about the world and how it works. They also have little life experience to make them question what they are told. Young children do not have the same thinking abilities as adults – and so they do not question things in the same way. So if a trusted adult tells a young child that the Tooth Fairy exists, then the child is likely to believe that this is true.

What about when a young child is told by a parent or a teacher that they are stupid? Or that they are a bad person? If this happens enough times then it makes perfect sense that the child begins to believe these things about themselves as absolutely true, just as they believe it when they are told that the Tooth Fairy exists.

Sometimes children are not told negative things about themselves directly but in less obvious ways. How about a child who is never praised by their parents? What might they begin to believe about themselves? In this case, a child might learn to believe 'I am no good' even though this has never been said to them directly. What about a child who has parents who are too busy with their own lives to pay them much attention? Might this child learn to believe 'I am not important'? Or a child who is physically abused and bullied, might they learn to believe 'I am weak and vulnerable'?

Although core beliefs often develop when we are young children, they can also develop later in life if we have had a traumatic experience. For instance, someone might learn to believe 'I am strong' when they are a young child but, if they are bullied or abused as an adult, this might change to the core belief 'I am weak'.

So, negative core beliefs (which lie at the heart of low self-esteem) develop for good reasons. They are our way of making sense of our life experiences, often at an age when we are too young to question our experiences or what we are told. But why don't our negative core beliefs tend to change as we get older, even if our experiences change? How come they tend to hang around even when we are adults?

Why does low self-esteem hang around?

There is an interesting fact about the human mind. When we believe something is true, we tend to look for reasons why it is true and we tend to ignore or twist evidence that does not fit with our beliefs. This is true for all of us – it is just the way our minds work.

Let's look again at Martin. One of Martin's negative core beliefs is 'I am stupid'. He developed this view of himself as a young child, seemingly based on good reasons: he struggled to read and write at primary school and noticed other children doing things he couldn't do. Martin also had a teacher who kept telling him to try harder. When he was 8 years old, he was diagnosed as being very short-sighted and started to wear glasses. Once this happened, his reading and writing caught up with the level achieved by his friends. However, by this point, his core belief 'I am stupid' was firmly rooted in his mind.

As an adult, Martin became very good at noticing reasons why this core belief was true. For instance, when he failed his first driving test. He also would sit and think about reasons why this belief must be true – and he would remember the critical comments from his former teacher. The more reasons Martin noticed to support his core belief, the more he believed it must be true. The picture below shows a vicious cycle that strengthens negative core beliefs:

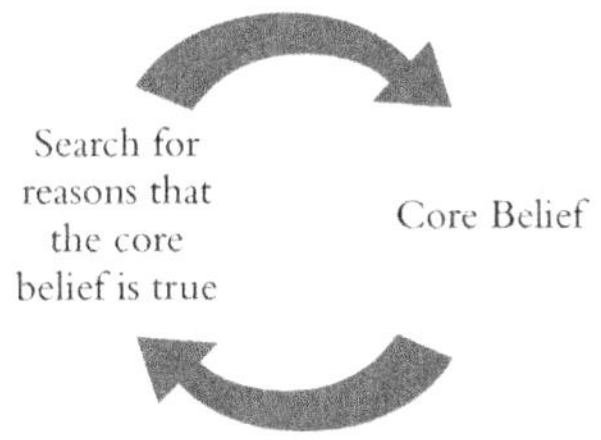

Martin

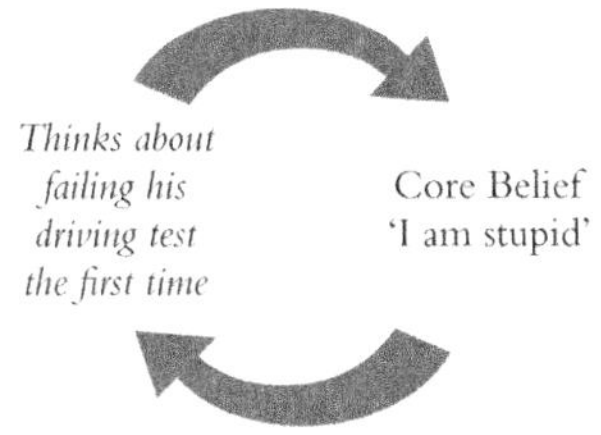

The other thing we all tend to do is ignore evidence that does not support our beliefs. For instance, Martin didn't change his core belief 'I am stupid' when he passed his driving test the second time around.

Another thing that some of us do is twist evidence to fit with our beliefs. So, rather than Martin taking pleasure from his friend telling him how much he valued their friendship, Martin would think 'my friends feel sorry for me because I am stupid'.

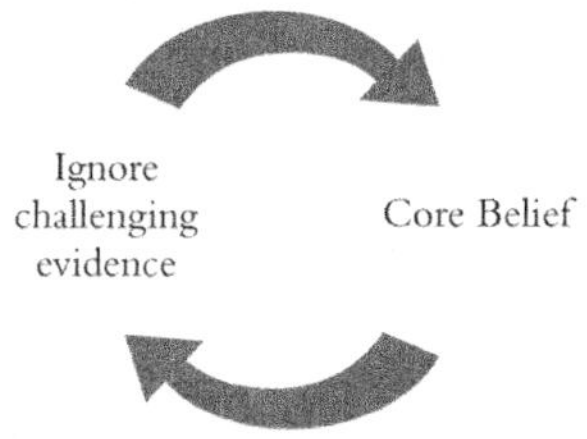

Martin

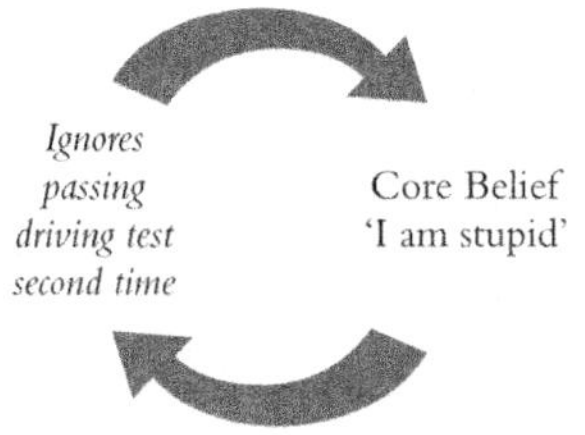

For all these reasons, once we develop a core belief about ourselves it tends to become stronger over time as we search for evidence that supports it, ignore evidence that does not support it and even twist evidence to make it fit. Martin's experiences are very common – and show that once we develop a negative view of ourselves it can be hard to change.

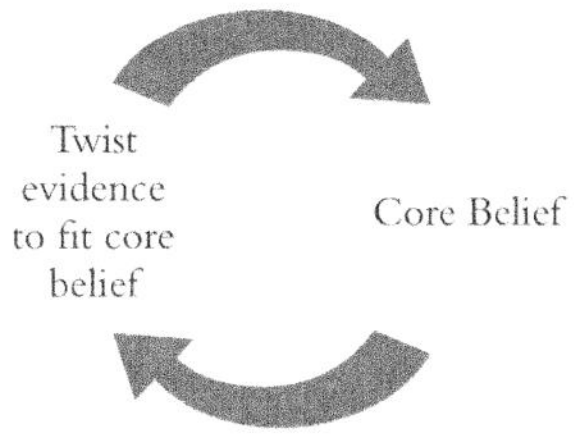

Martin

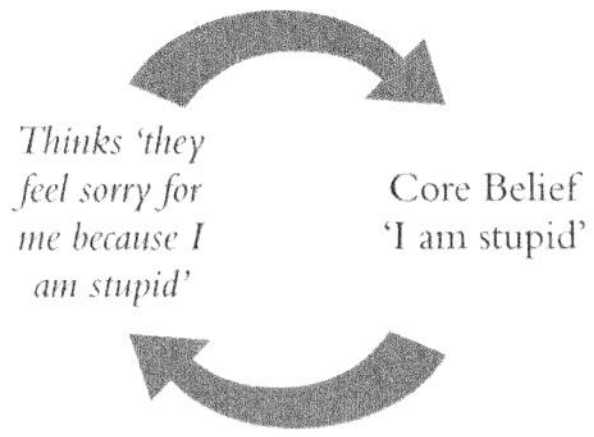

Low self-esteem and rules for living

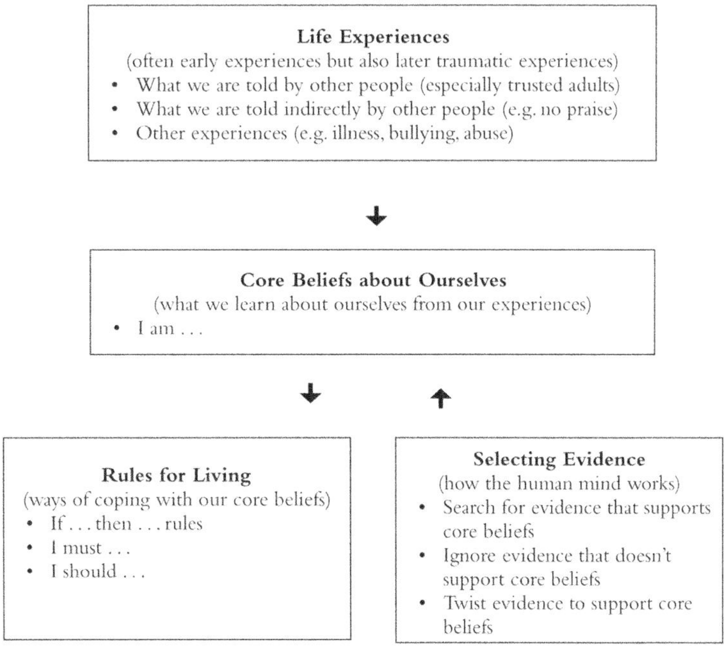

Figure 5: What is low self-esteem?

Another reason why low self-esteem tends to persist is that we develop ways of coping with our negative core beliefs – and this can stop us from questioning their accuracy. These ways of coping with core beliefs are sometimes called 'rules for living' – that is to say, the rules we have for living our lives based on the apparent truth of our core beliefs.

We can usually write down our rules for living as 'if ... then...' statements, or as statements about what we *must* or *should* do. One 'rule for living' that Martin had developed – a rule to try to cope with his core belief that he is stupid – was: 'If I don't try then I won't prove how stupid I am.'

Martin figured out that if he didn't try to succeed then he couldn't fail – and thus no one would notice how stupid he was. So he didn't bother applying to go to college, and he turned down the chance of applying for a job he was interested in. Martin used the fact that he didn't have qualifications and that he didn't have a job as evidence to support his core belief. This is how rules for living work – they are our way of coping with our core beliefs but these ways of coping often strengthen our negative beliefs about ourselves.

What is low self-esteem? A summary so far

The diagram in Figure 5 summarizes the ideas we have looked at so far. We learn about ourselves from our life experiences (and usually from our earliest experiences). Once we have formed ideas about who we are, these ideas tend to become stronger through our rules for living and through the ways that we select evidence. But what has all this got to do with hearing voices?

Low self-esteem and hearing voices

Feeling distressed at hearing voices and having low self-esteem usually go together. A recent study found that low self-esteem was very common among people who were distressed by hearing voices. The study also found that low self-esteem was linked to feeling depressed.[3] So why is it so common for people who are distressed by hearing voices to also have low self-esteem?

Life experiences, low self-esteem and distressing voices

We have already seen that low self-esteem is to do with having strong, negative ideas about ourselves (core beliefs). We have also seen that we learn negative ideas about ourselves for good reasons – because of the experiences we have had. So why are distressing voices linked to low self-esteem?

---

3 See Fannon, D., Hayward, P., Thompson, N., Green, N., Surguladze, S. & Wykes, T. (2009). 'The self or the voice? Relative contributions of self-esteem and voice appraisal in persistent auditory hallucinations'. Schizophrenia Research, 112, 174–180

People who are distressed by hearing voices are very likely to have had particularly difficult early life experiences. Research studies have found that the majority of people who hear distressing voices have experienced abuse as children. Although childhood abuse is common for people experiencing mental health problems more generally, childhood abuse is especially common among people who are distressed by hearing voices. Abuse might be physical or sexual. Abuse can also involve neglect of one form or another.

Experts from many different areas all agree that children can never be responsible in any way for being the victim of abuse. Unfortunately, however, it is common for children who are abused to blame themselves. This might be because they are told they are to blame (which we know is not true). If a child blames themselves then they may develop core beliefs such as 'I am a bad person' or 'I am weak and vulnerable' or 'I am no good'. We have already seen how, once these core beliefs are there, they tend to become stronger as we search for reasons why they must be true and ignore reasons why they are not true. So, one reason why low self-esteem and distressing voices often go together is that people who are distressed by voices are more likely than not to have had some very difficult and traumatic life experiences.

Not everyone who hears voices has been abused as a child. Some people who are distressed by voices may have had other kinds of difficult experiences in their lives such as being bullied at school or not being praised much by either parents or teachers. As we saw earlier, these kinds of difficult life experience can lead to us believing negative things about ourselves such as 'I am unlikeable' or 'I am not worthwhile'. Just as we saw earlier, once we begin to believe these things about ourselves, we start to look for reasons why they are true and to dismiss any evidence that does not fit with our beliefs.

It is important to remember that not all people who are distressed by hearing voices have low self-esteem or have had difficult life experiences. Although this is true for most people who hear distressing voices, it is not true for everyone.

Low self-esteem and beliefs about voices

At the end of Chapter 1 we saw that people who are distressed by hearing voices are quite likely to believe that the voices are powerful, controlling or are trying to cause harm. Is there a link between these kinds of beliefs about voices and low self-esteem?

Let's look again at the ABC model we first saw in Chapter 1.

Figure 6 is the same as Figure 2 shown in Chapter 1; the only difference is that 'core beliefs about myself' have been added and there is now an arrow drawn between 'core beliefs about myself' and 'beliefs and thoughts about voices'. This shows how core beliefs about ourselves can directly influence the beliefs and thoughts we have about the voices.

Let's return to Martin's story. Now that we have looked at core beliefs and how they develop, what core beliefs might we expect Martin to have about himself? In his life story (see section entitled "How do people react to voices?") we were told that Martin was beaten by his stepfather, so it is no surprise to learn that Martin came to the conclusion 'I am weak and vulnerable' about himself. He was then bullied while in the army, which made him believe even more strongly that he was weak and vulnerable. What about when Martin was a young child and his father left and he never saw him again? How might that have affected Martin? Is it understandable that Martin believed he was no good and not worth anything?

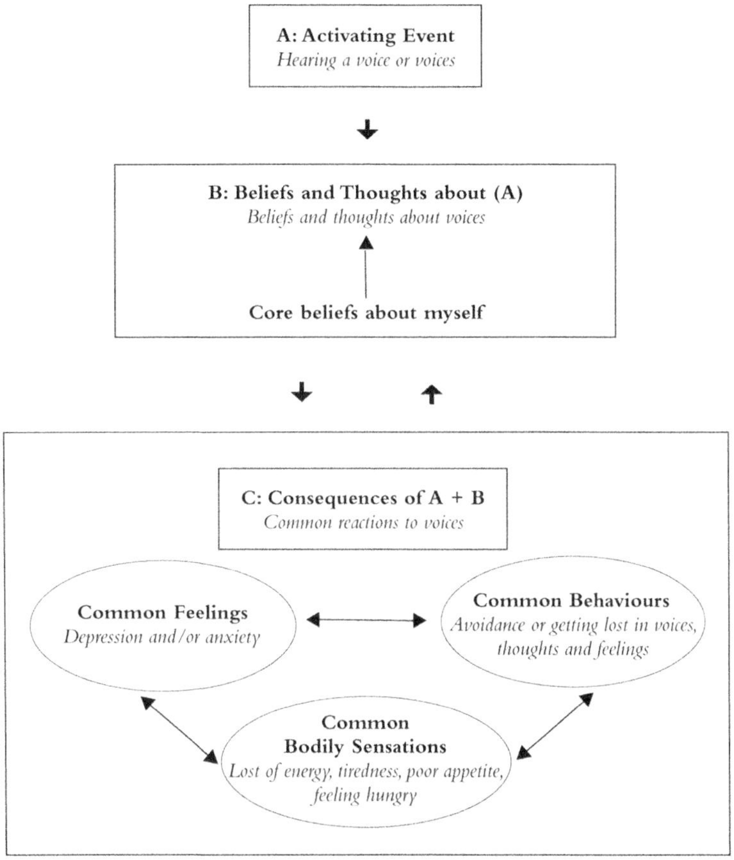

Figure 6: A Cognitive Behaviour Therapy approach to understanding voices – the ABC model

Looking at Martin's story we can understand how he came to have these negative core beliefs about himself:

- I am weak and vulnerable
- I am no good
- I'm not worth anything

If you read Martin's story again, what do *you* think? Do you agree that Martin is weak and no good? Or do you see Martin in a different way to how he sees himself? These core beliefs are not the truth about Martin, but he believes they are true because that is what his early life experience taught him.

Let's turn now to what Martin believes about the voices he hears. When we look at Figure 7, we see he believes:

- Voices speak the truth (he believes they are right when they say he is no good and that no one will ever love him)
- Voices have the power to harm him

By putting together Martin's negative core beliefs, and his beliefs about the voices, it is now fairly clear that what Martin believes about himself as a person influences what he believes about the voices he hears. Martin believes he is no good, and he believes it when the voices tell him he is no good. Martin also believes it when the voices tell him that no one will ever love him – because he has the core belief that he is unlovable. Added to this, Martin believes that the voices have the power to harm him, which seems to fit with his core belief that he is weak and vulnerable.

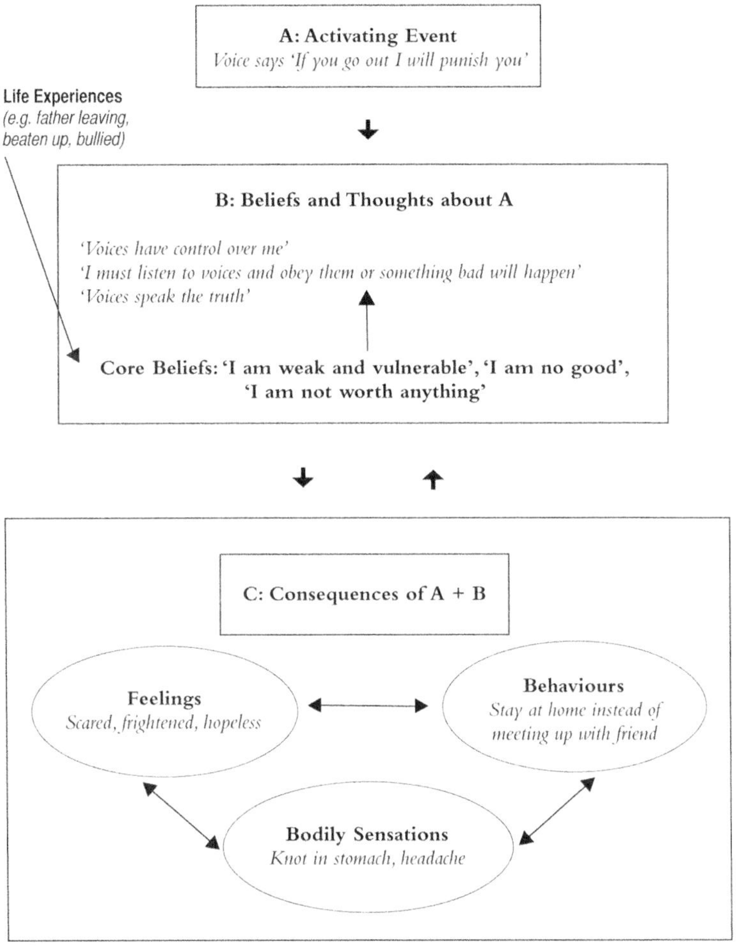

Figure 7: Martin

Figure 7 looks at how Martin's core beliefs were his way of making sense of his early experiences. It also shows how one of his core beliefs directly influenced how he thought about the voices he heard. When a voice said, 'if you go out I will punish you', Martin believed the voice had control over him and that he must obey it: this is due to his core belief that he is weak and vulnerable.

Summary

In this chapter, we have seen that feeling distressed by voices is often associated with low self-esteem. This is because, in both cases, negative beliefs are at the root of the problem. When it comes to low self-esteem, core beliefs are about viewing ourselves negatively. When it comes to feeling distressed by voices, negative beliefs are usually about voices being powerful, controlling and intending harm. In this chapter, we have suggested that negative core beliefs about ourselves (that usually develop in early childhood) can have a direct influence on how we think about voices. This means that if we can change our view of ourselves by letting go of strongly held negative core beliefs, and by acknowledging more positive aspects of ourselves, then this might directly influence how we think and feel about voices. Later, in Chapter 6, we will look at how we can begin to change core beliefs about ourselves in this way.

Key points

- Negative core beliefs are 'I am...' statements about ourselves that seem completely true and lie at the heart of low self-esteem.
- Negative core beliefs are our way of making sense of difficult life experiences (often from early childhood).

- Although negative core beliefs are our way of making sense of difficult experiences, they are rarely true.
- Negative core beliefs persist because we tend to look for reasons why they are true and ignore evidence that they are not true.
- People distressed by hearing voices are particularly likely to have had difficult life experiences and this is why they are very likely to have negative beliefs about themselves.
- Negative core beliefs can directly influence beliefs about voices. If someone has the core belief 'I am weak' then they are likely to believe that voices are powerful and controlling.
- If we can overcome low self-esteem, this can be a step towards overcoming distressing voices.

3

Relationships with voices and other people

In Chapter 2 we learnt how our early life experiences can shape the development of our self-esteem. We saw that people distressed by hearing voices often have low self-esteem, which can play a key role in maintaining the distress that the voices cause. Low self-esteem can also affect the relationships that we have with other people. For example, in Chapter 2 we saw how Martin's core beliefs about being weak and vulnerable led him to obey his voice and stay at home – denying him opportunities to spend time with friends. This chapter will consider the relationships we have with other people and how these relationships might influence the way that we respond to hearing voices.

What do we mean by relationship?

What is a relationship? When we talk about relationships we usually mean something that happens between two people. Within a relationship, people are likely to spend time together and influence each other. It is worth noting that, in the twenty-first century, relationships do not always mean that people have to be in the same place: people can meet, get to know each other and hang out on Facebook, virtual worlds such as Second Life, chat rooms, etc.

We might expect that having a relationship with someone should be pleasurable; something that we look forward to and welcome. When relationships work well, we are likely to experience a lot of giving and taking within these relationships, and to feel good about ourselves when we are together. For many people, the majority of their relationships are like this. However, we also know that some relationships can be difficult and a source of distress and pain. In these relationships we may be bullied by the other person, not listened to, or we might feel hurt and abused. These relationships can be especially damaging if we feel trapped within them and think we cannot escape. One key feature of difficult relationships can be the lack of give and take. When this happens, the person who feels distressed is likely to feel they have little say in the relationship.

How do we understand relationships?

Social scientists have been trying to understand relationships for a long time. Much of their work has focused upon the give and take within relationships: if someone behaves in a certain way towards the other person, how does the other person respond? An interesting question is whether certain types of behaviour are more or less likely to lead to similar or different responses, e.g. will behaving aggressively cause the other person to be aggressive in response? Or, will behaving aggressively cause the other person to feel afraid and respond by backing off? Will a request for some time apart be accepted or will it be seen as a threat and cause the other person in the relationship to become more clingy?

In response to these questions, psychiatrist John Birtchnell has suggested that we can think about relationships in two main ways: in terms of 'power' and 'closeness'. Let's look at these ideas in a little more detail.

Power and relationships

When it comes to relationships, 'power' means how much influence one person has over the other person and how they use it. We can probably all think of relationships where there are different levels of power, e.g. bosses have more power than their workers, parents have more power than their children. If power is used in a positive way, someone may use their power to help another person, and the other person may gratefully accept their help. However, if the more powerful person uses their power in a negative way, they may try to dominate the other person and push them around. The person who is being dominated may then either accept being pushed around – and behave quite submissively – or they may try to fight back. All these ways of responding will mean that it is likely that the powerful person continues to behave in the same way. See Figure 8 for an illustration of the way power can work in relationships.

Closeness and relationships

John Birtchnell suggests that closeness refers to both the *physical* closeness and the *emotional* closeness of two people in a relationship. If one person wants to get closer, and behaves in ways that makes the other person want to get closer, then the distance between them is likely to reduce (they will spend more time together and feel closer emotionally). Likewise, if one person wants some space and time apart, and requests this in a positive way, the other person is likely to respect their wish and back off for a while. However, closeness in relationships can also be expressed in a negative way. Someone may feel the other person is trying to get too close (it feels intrusive) or they may feel the other person is becoming too distant. If someone in a relationship behaves in a clingy way, then the other person may want to withdraw and get away from them. See Figure 9 for an illustration of how closeness can work in relationships.

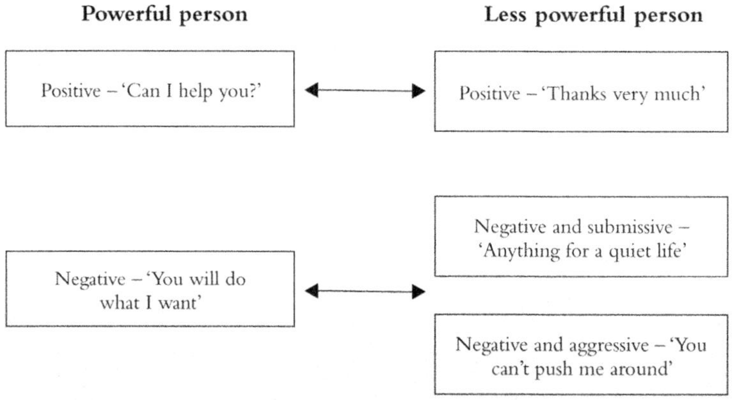

Figure 8: Positive and negative use of power in relationships

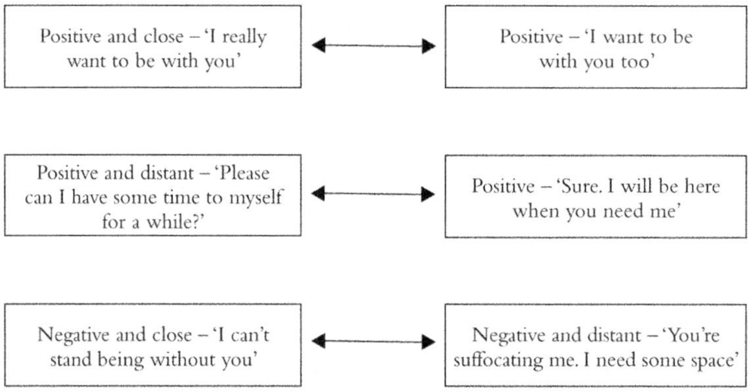

Figure 9: Positive and negative closeness in relationships

When we consider relationships in terms of power and closeness, the two-way process between people is apparent. The behaviour of one person in a relationship can influence the behaviour of the other, and vice versa.

So, what has all this got to do with voices? Let us first look briefly at the question of whether or not people who hear voices 'have relationships' with those voices.

Can we have relationships with voices?

We asked people who heard distressing voices about whether or not they had relationships with their voices. Many of these people spoke of having two-way conversations with their voices. For instance, Donna said:

> *I suppose it's two-way, in that we have conversations. I tell them [the voices] to go away, they tell me they're not going to; they ask me to do things, I tell them I'm not going to ... and so we have conversations in that way, so, in that way it's two-way.*

Norman describes the dialogue he has with his deceased mother's voice:

> *She asks me how my day is going and I tell her what I've done and what I'm doing, then I ask how she's been today, what she's done.*

Research has shown that many people have two-way conversations like this with their voices. So perhaps the idea of having a relationship with voices is not such a strange idea.

The rest of this chapter will look in more detail at how relationships with voices are affected by power and closeness. We will also look at the possible similarities between 'real world' relationships and relationships with voices.

Power and closeness in relationships with voices

As we saw in Chapter 1, some people who hear voices do not feel upset or distressed by them and the voices do not have a big influence on their lives. In such cases, people tend to see themselves as having enough power in their relationship with the voices, and they can control the distance between themselves and the voice.

Distressing voices, on the other hand, tend to be seen as very powerful, and much more powerful than the people who hear them. This is a very common view among those who hear distressing voices. The voices are often regarded as using their power in a negative way to try to dominate us, intrude upon our privacy by being too close, push us around, command us to do harmful things, or bully us with insults and put-downs. Sean describes how his voices disrespect his need for space and distance by intruding upon his thinking:

> *...every thought I'm thinking, they're hearing and they're saying to me, 'well, that thought was wrong and you should change it like this...'*

Ulrika describes the way her voices try to control her:

> *...the voices try to control my life in every possible way, for example, they try to twist the truth on some level, so I think that they're playing a kind of little game with my life and try to affect who is my friend and who I'm going to get close to...*

You might like to rate how powerful and close you find your voice(s) by answering the questions in the two questionnaires below. If you hear more than one voice, try to rate your main voice. Add your scores for each scale. The higher your total score, the more powerful or close you think your voice is. Remember that viewing voices as powerful and too close is not unusual. In Part Three of this book, we will look at ways of taking power away from the voices and how we can feel more powerful even when the voices are around.

Figure 10: Rating the power of your voice (Items taken from the Voice and You questionnaire, Hayward et al., 2008)

My voice tries to get the better of me

Nearly always true (score 3)

____

____

____

Quite Often True (score 2)

Sometimes true (score 1)

Rarely true (score 0)

My voice makes me feel useless

Nearly always true (score 3)

Quite Often True (score 2)

Sometimes true (score 1)

Rarely true (score 0)

My voice tries to make me out to be stupid

Nearly always true (score 3)

Quite Often True (score 2)

Sometimes true (score 1)

Rarely true (score 0)

My voice wants things done his/her way

Nearly always true (score 3)

Quite Often True (score 2)

Sometimes true (score 1)

Rarely true (score 0)

My voice makes hurtful remarks to me

Nearly always true (score 3)

Quite Often True (score 2)

Sometimes true (score 1)

Rarely true (score 0)

My voice constantly reminds me of my failings

Nearly always true (score 3)

Quite Often True (score 2)

Sometimes true (score 1)

Rarely true (score 0)

My voice does not give me credit for the good things I do

Nearly always true (score 3)

Quite Often True (score 2)

Sometimes true (score 1)

Rarely true (score 0)

The power rating for my voice is _____/21

Figure 11: Rating the closeness of your voice (Items taken from the Voice and You questionnaire, Hayward et al., 2008)

My voice finds it hard to allow me to have time away from him/her

Nearly always true (score 3)

Quite Often True (score 2)

Sometimes true (score 1)

Rarely true (score 0)

My voice dislikes spending time on his/her own

Nearly always true (score 3)

Quite Often True (score 2)

Sometimes true (score 1)

Rarely true (score 0)

My voice tries to accompany me when I go out

Nearly always true (score 3)

Quite Often True (score 2)

Sometimes true (score 1)

Rarely true (score 0)

My voice dislikes it when I exclude him/her by showing an interest in other people

Nearly always true (score 3)

Quite Often True (score 2)

Sometimes true (score 1)

Rarely true (score 0)

My voice does not let me have time to myself

Nearly always true (score 3)

Quite Often True (score 2)

Sometimes true (score 1)

Rarely true (score 0)

The closeness rating for my voice is _____/15

Responding to voices by trying to escape

When we view our distressing voices as powerful, or too close, we may understandably feel a desire to try to escape from them and to create some distance between ourselves and the voices. Distraction techniques such as listening to music, humming or talking to other people can be quite successful on a temporary basis and we will look at these techniques in more detail in Chapter 4. Trying to escape and create distance between ourselves and our voice is understandable in the face of a dominating and intrusive bully, and may lead to some relief in the short term. However, as this tends to be a *forced* reaction to the voice – in other words, we feel we have no other option – rather than being an *active* choice, such a response may do little to change our relationship with the voice in the long term. If we remind ourselves of what we learnt in Chapter 2, about how low self-esteem can often go hand in hand with hearing distressing voices, then it becomes clear that responding in a passive way to voices is likely to strengthen any views that we have about ourselves as being weak (see Figure 12 below).

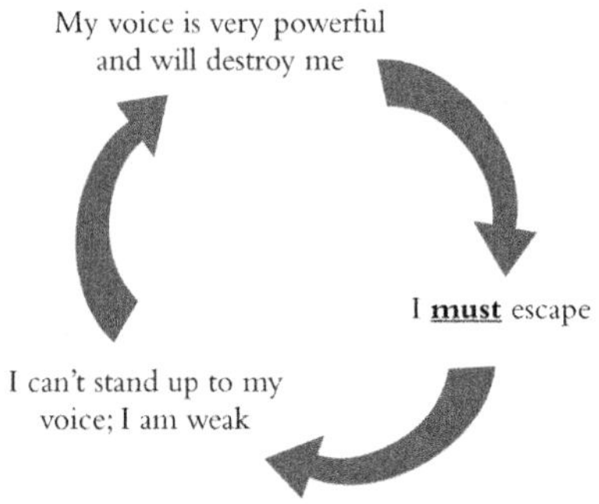

Figure 12: Responses to voices that maintain low self-esteem

Responding to voices by fighting back

Another common reaction to hearing a powerful voice that feels too close is to fight back. For example, shouting at the voice, swearing or hurling insults at it. Let's look at how Donna describes the way that she fights back against her voice:

> *Therapist: When you say you try to fight your voices, how do you try to do that?*
>
> *Donna: Well, I say 'go away I'm not listening', or 'shut up' and if they swear at me I swear back at them. So I tell them I'm not listening, but they just demand that I listen.*
>
> *Therapist: So, they're not that responsive to your attempts, then?*
>
> *Donna: No, they don't go away when I tell them to, they're persistent.*

Like the passive response described earlier, this type of aggressive response might offer some relief in the short term but it may also have the opposite effect – as responding aggressively can sometimes result in an even more aggressive reaction from the voice. If the voice shouts more loudly and is more insulting, this may have the effect of strengthening any negative core beliefs you might have about being weak.

Responding to voices by giving in

A third possible reaction to powerful and intrusive voices is to give in to them. For some of us, this may be a gut reaction to a very powerful voice that seems overwhelming. For others, giving in may be a sign of feeling hopeless – and that we have given up trying to fight back. If you have been trying to escape from your voice or fight it for a long time without much success, or things have got worse, giving in might offer some relief from unsuccessfully trying to get the better of the voice. Some people who hear voices say that giving in can mean an easier life. However, just as attempting to escape your voices, or fighting back, can have a negative effect on your self-esteem in the long term, so too can giving in, as this can strengthen any core beliefs you may hold about being weak.

Martin's responses to his voice

Martin has tried all three ways of responding: escaping, fighting back and giving in. Initially, he gave in and did what his voice said. But after a while he became concerned about the consequences of obeying the voice, as it started to ask him to do extreme things such as harming himself. This led Martin to try distraction – listening to music. This worked for a while, but nothing really changed. As a result, Martin became frustrated and began to respond aggressively to the voice. This was not helpful at all, as the voice just shouted back more loudly and more aggressively. So, Martin has ended up where he started, by giving in to the voice and obeying its commands – but not fully obeying if the things he is being told to do are too extreme.

Responding differently to voices

In the last section we focused on the two-way relationships that we can have with the voices we hear. However, these relationships are often imbalanced, as powerful and intrusive voices tend to call most of the shots. This pattern of one-way relating is common with distressing voices, and often leaves us to conclude that no relationship exists between the voice and ourselves:

> *Ulrika: I've said to the voices many times that 'there's you or me but no we'.*

If a proper relationship did exist, surely it would be two-way? We have suggested that a relationship can and does exist between a person and the voices they hear, but by trying to escape the voice, or by giving in to it, we are relating in a passive way and may have no sense that we can influence the relationship. However, if we respond more actively to the voice, this may provoke it to being even more aggressive. If the relationship with the voice is to become more balanced and less distressing, it can be very helpful to become more assertive in our responses. Being assertive means not reacting passively to voices but it also means not acting aggressively. This sounds easier said than done in the face of a bombardment from a powerful and intrusive voice, so we will spend time in Chapter 7 looking at how to be assertive towards voices. In the meantime, using Figure 13, let us consider what we have learnt about relationships so far.

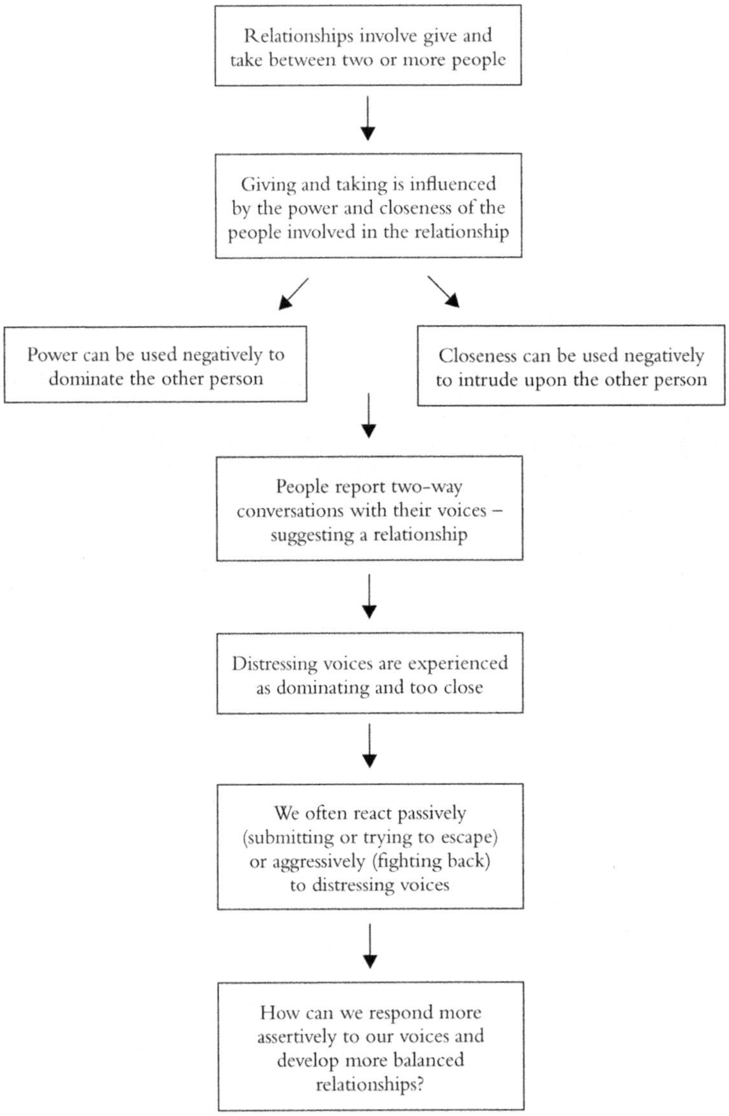

Figure 13: How we develop relationships with our voices

What about my relationships with friends and family?

If distressing voices are viewed as powerful and too close, and provoke us into reacting passively or aggressively, are all our relationships like this? Do we have similar relationships with the people in our social lives? Or are the relationships we have with our voices different to the relationships we have with our friends and family?

Recall from Chapter 1 the findings that we looked at in relation to Romme and Escher's survey of 450 people who heard voices: the survey revealed that many people were able to cope with their voices. Those who coped with their voices had a number of things in common:

- They were likely to be married.
- They perceived themselves to be well-supported by other people.
- They were likely to have someone they could confide in about their voices.

This list suggests that the people who are able to cope with their voices have positive relationships with friends and family. These positive relationships provide many opportunities to receive support from people whose opinions are valued and trusted, and might include the possibility that the voices can be talked about openly. Thus, the voices can be explored and questioned.

If positive relationships with friends and family can have a beneficial effect upon our relationship with voices, what happens if relationships with friends and family are negative? A research study conducted in 2004 by Max Birchwood and colleagues asked 125 people who heard distressing voices to respond about their relationships with friends and family, and their relationships with the voices. People reported a lack of power and status within *all* these relationships, suggesting that relationships with people in the 'real world' are similar to relationships with voices. Many people also said that their relationships with friends and family influenced their relationship with the voices (rather than the other way around). So it seems that there can be an important connection between the kind of relationships we have with people and those we have with voices – and that it is the relationships we have with people that can influence those we develop with voices.

If positive relationships with friends and family can have a positive effect on our relationship with voices, and negative relationships likewise have a negative influence, is it possible to have a positive experience in one area and a negative experience in the other? We all have a strong need and desire to be in relationships. If our relationships with friends and family are negative, and if none of our needs and desires for relationships are met in the 'real world', could our relationship with voices be the next best thing? Do some of us escape from the difficult relationships in our social lives into a relatively more predictable and safer world of our voices? Research suggests that this does sometimes happen, and as the relationship with voices becomes more and more important it can become difficult to give it up. This is the case with Norman's experience:

> *I haven't got many friends ... so the only thing I can stay very close to are the voices and I do stay very close to them.*

Some people have described relationships with their voices as being a close and positive experience, whereas relationships in their social lives were described as less important. Some people with more difficult social lives appeared to find solace in the voices, which sometimes seemed to fulfil a 'friendship' role. This is illustrated by Russell's comment:

> *I haven't told anyone this for years, I made a little joke with the consultant in the hospital and said if they [the voices] stopped I'd quite miss them. They're almost like part of me and sometimes when I don't hear them I think 'where are the voices?'*

Comparing Martin's and Sarah's stories

We saw in Chapter 1 that Martin and Sarah had similar voice-hearing experiences as both had heard the voice of an abuser from the past. However, their responses to the voices were quite different: Martin was distressed by a voice that he viewed as very powerful, and he did what the voice told him; Sarah was less distressed by her voice, as experience had suggested that the voice was not very powerful, so she didn't follow its orders.

In terms of relationships, both Martin and Sarah hear voices that behave in powerful and intrusive ways. The important difference is in their response. Martin responds passively by doing what the voice tells him. He thinks that he has no say within the relationship and thus gives in to the wishes of the voice. There is a clear link between his past relationships with powerful and intrusive family members (father) and friends (colleagues in the army), his negative core beliefs about himself, his passive response to the voice, and the implications for current and future relationships with family and friends (i.e. staying at home instead of meeting up with people).

Figure 14, overleaf, adds these issues to the diagram of Martin's experience that we saw earlier, to show that the impact of negative relationships flows from Martin's past through to his future. What might happen if Martin were able to change the way he responds within relationships with people and with voices? In Chapter 7 we will look at ways of responding differently in relationships, and then see what difference this has made to Martin.

Sarah takes a more active approach than Martin by choosing not to do what the voice tells her to do. She thinks that she has a choice about her role within the relationship, and chooses to relate in an assertive way that is consistent with the facts about her voice – it has not hurt her in the past fifteen years, so probably won't be able to do so in the future. There are clear links here between Sarah's past positive relationships with family and friends, her positive core beliefs about herself, her assertive response to the voice, and the positive relationships she has with friends and family. Figure 15 adds these issues to the diagram of Sarah's experience that we saw earlier, and shows that, just as with Martin, the impact of relationships flows from Sarah's past through to her present and future.

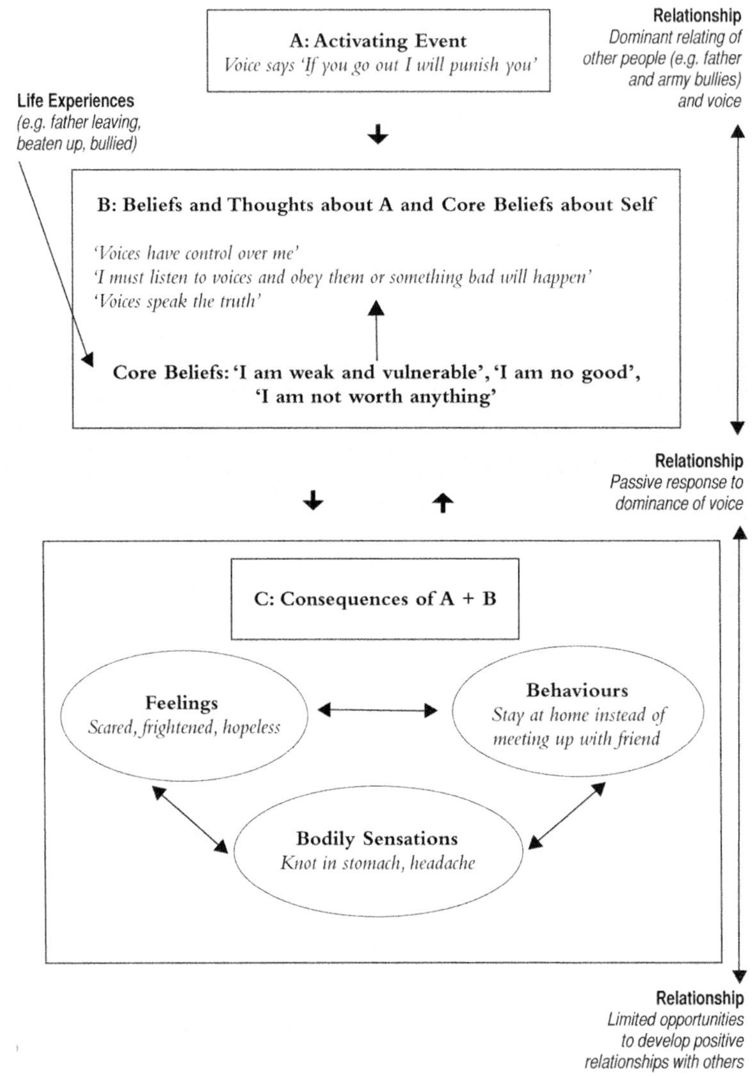

Figure 14: Martin's relationships

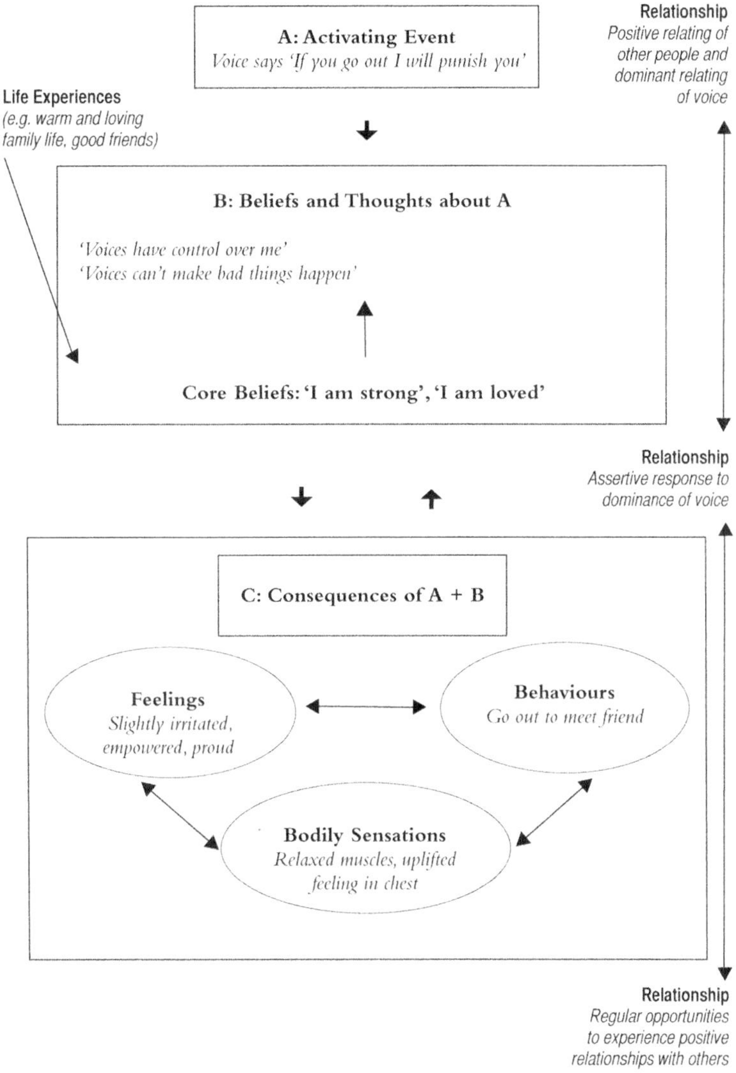

Figure 15: Sarah's relationships

Summary

In this chapter we have seen how our relationships with our voices can mirror our relationships with friends and family. What is most interesting about this realization is what it means for *changing* our relationships: positively changing how we respond to friends and family – trying to develop more assertive and balanced relationships – may have a knock-on effect of changing our relationships with voices. These possibilities for changing how we respond in our relationships will be explored further in Chapter 7.

Key points

- Relationships involve give and take between two or more people.
- Giving and taking is influenced by the power and closeness of the people involved.
- Power and closeness can be used negatively by one person to dominate and intrude upon the other person.
- We often have two-way conversations with our voices – so we are probably having a relationship of sorts.
- Distressing voices are usually experienced as powerful and intrusive.
- We often respond passively or aggressively to distressing voices.
- Our past and present relationships with family and friends can influence our relationships with voices.
- Changing our relationships with voices will have a positive knock-on effect on relationships with friends and family – and vice versa.

Part Two

Responding Differently to Distressing Voices

In Part One of this book we considered three key areas:

- Voices – what they are, what can cause them and how they make us feel.
- Ourselves – how we view ourselves and how this can impact on the way voices make us feel.
- Relationships – how we have two-way relationships with the people in our social lives *and* with our voices, and how these relationships can become imbalanced and cause us distress.

In Part Three we will discover how to make changes in each of these areas:

- Chapter 5 looks at changing the beliefs we might hold about our voices.
- Chapter 6 considers how to change the negative beliefs that we might have about ourselves.
- Chapter 7 explores ways of changing the relationships that we have with our voices and the people in our social lives.

Before thinking about change – as addressed in Part Three – in the next chapter we look at different ways of coping with distressing voices. If *change* is about taking steps to make things better (reducing the distress caused by voices), then *coping* is more about taking steps to stop things from getting worse (stopping the distress caused by voices from increasing). This difference between coping and change may seem unimportant, but it may in fact create some stepping stones towards us being in a better place with our voices. Some of us may find it helpful to start by developing a few ways of coping with our voices. When we have found ways of coping, then we can either stop there, or use our new-found confidence to try to make some changes. Others among us will have the confidence to dive straight in to making changes. However, there is no right place to start, so please start in the place that makes most sense to you.

4

Coping with voices

Trying to understand our voices can help reduce the confusion and distress that they cause, so it is worth trying to be as clear as possible when we talk about them. As already discussed, we use the term voices when there doesn't seem to be anybody actually saying the things we are hearing. This can be very puzzling, at least at first. We might try to work out who is speaking, and we might ask other people if they can hear the voices. However, although the nature of voices is that they are something only you can hear, it is worth checking with someone you can trust (such as a family member or friend, or a nurse, doctor or therapist) if you are not sure if other people can hear what you're hearing. This can be a bit embarrassing if the voice is saying bad things about you – but it is better to know than just to guess whether other people can hear it or not.

Martin

Martin hears his stepfather insulting him and putting him down. He asked his sister if she could hear their stepfather speaking. She said 'no', so Martin knew for sure that this was a voice.

If what you are hearing is attributable to voices – that is, auditory hallucinations – others will tell you that they can't hear them. So what do you think might be causing them? It may be clear to you what the cause is – it might be related to other things happening in your life or things that have happened in the past – and this is something that you can discuss with others. However, many people are uncertain about how voices start and what brings them on. You might want to go back and look at Chapter 1, which describes the origin of voices in more detail. Why do you hear voices and others don't? And then comes the most important thing – what can you do to cope with them?

Some questions about voices:

1. Are they just like someone speaking or shouting?
2. Where do they seem to come from?
3. Do other people hear them?
4. If they don't hear them, why do you think that is?
5. What could be causing your voices?
6. How can you cope with them most effectively?

Hearing voices can be distressing even if we have a good understanding of them. Thus developing effective ways of coping with them can be very helpful.

Sometimes voices can interfere with our coping mechanisms and can tell us not to do things that may otherwise actually help. They can also command us to do things that are not good for us, and we might even find that voices threaten us if we don't do what they say. If you find that this is the case then it would be a good idea to talk to someone who can help, such as a mental health professional or doctor, or maybe someone who is able to understand and offer support such as a close family member or a good friend. They may be able to help you work out what is going on and support you to resist doing what the voice is commanding you to do. There are also a number of techniques that people have learnt to use in order to try to cope with voices. These divide broadly into three groups, which involve using meaningful activities to improve coping by providing positive alternatives to listening to the voices: stress management – helping you to relax; social measures – other people who can help; mental health treatments and interventions – professionals can also help you to cope with hearing voices. While the voices may continue in the background when using these techniques, they will nevertheless become less prominent and should feel easier to manage, even if only for a while. Let's look at each of these techniques in more detail.

Stress management

This involves carrying out activities that help to soothe us, activities that can ease the tension that can make voices worse. These activities are fairly simple. They can involve a bit of effort, which we may not feel we have the energy for, but sometimes they actually mean doing less, allowing us to relax.

One method is to try soothing ourselves by taking a warm bath or having a sauna (some local leisure centres have sauna facilities). Bubble bath or aromatherapy oils may improve the experience – pleasant smells can increase your sense of relaxation. The voices may tell you that you don't deserve to relax, but what do they know? Who doesn't deserve to relax from time to time?

Many people who hear voices find that peaceful experiences such as carrying out a relaxation exercise can be very beneficial and enable them to cope better. Breathing exercises or progressive muscle relaxation (PMR) – working round your body tensing and relaxing each muscle in turn – can feel really good and help you to overcome stress and anxious feelings: gentle rhythmic tensing and relaxing of parts of the body is something that can be done without fuss but which can calm us and get us back in control of a situation. A PMR exercise is described in more detail below.

Progressive muscle relaxation (PMR) exercise

There is one basic movement that you will use at every stage of the exercise, which is as follows:

Tense your muscles, but do not strain, and concentrate on the sensation of tension. Work round your body, bit by bit, up one side and then down the other. Each time you tense, hold this for about five seconds and then let go of the tension for ten to fifteen seconds. Discover how your muscles feel when you relax them.

PMR involves doing this action for each of the muscle groups throughout your body. It is important to breathe slowly and regularly throughout the exercise, and it should be done in a place that is comfortable and where you won't be disturbed, e.g. on your bed or in an armchair. Focus on each part of your body in turn, as follows:

• Feet – pull your toes back, tense the muscles in your feet. Relax and repeat.

• Legs – straighten your legs and point your toes towards your face. Concentrate on calf muscles first, then thigh muscles. Relax, let your legs go limp and repeat.

• Abdomen – tense your stomach muscles by pulling them in and up – as if preparing to receive a punch. Relax and repeat.

• Back – arch your back. Relax and repeat.

- Shoulders/neck – shrug your shoulders as hard as you can, bringing them up and in. Press your head back. Relax and repeat.
- Arms – stretch out your arms and hands. Relax, let your arms hang limp and repeat.
- Face – tense your forehead and jaw. Lower your eyebrows and bite hard. Relax and repeat.
- Whole body – tense your entire body. Hold the tension for a few seconds. Relax and repeat.

(This exercise is adapted from *Overcoming Anxiety,* by Helen Kennerley)

We have mentioned in previous chapters that music can offer some temporary relief from voices. Music can be peaceful or energetic and both types can help us to relax. Depending on your taste – whether gentle orchestral music, love songs or heavy rock – music can help you unwind and can reduce the tension that tends to make voices worse. Getting absorbed in music can feel good and sometimes has the effect of drowning out the voices – although the voices may try to rise above it. If the voices do this, try to let them just wash over you: see if you can tune in to the music and tune out the voices. Spoken word (for example, audiobooks or radio programmes) can also work very well, particularly if they can get our attention and keep it for a while. Using headphones and an iPod or MP3 player can make the experience more effective – and also avoid our neighbours and family complaining!

Taking regular exercise can be very helpful as we know that there are proven links between good physical health and good mental health. Even if you don't particularly enjoy doing exercise, there is likely to be something that you don't mind doing – for example, a half-hour walk in the morning, or some gentle exercises to a DVD at home – and the benefits of committing yourself to doing exercise regularly are likely to be substantial. If it has been a while since you last did any exercise and you feel daunted at the prospect, then choose a time to do it that is convenient: for example, your lunch-hour, or early mornings. If you're going to the gym for the first time in a while, go when it is likely to be quiet. You also might want to try gradually building up the intensity of your exercise regime, but try to make it regular. If it is also a social occasion – meeting or going with somebody – then this can help motivate us but is not essential. Sometimes going alone is less stressful and more flexible, at least when you're getting started. If you want to go with someone, see whether there is a family member or friend who will go with you, or it may be possible for someone from mental health services to go with you, or a nurse or social worker if you see one, alternatively a support worker or maybe a volunteer befriender – it is well worth asking, if you think it might help.

Another good form of stress management is to retreat to a quiet place to find peace and a bit of tranquillity – but let your family know or they may start worrying, which might then interfere with your attempts to get peace and quiet if they keep checking on your whereabouts. Some people take this further and actually join short retreats, where they find peace and quiet and are able to use their time for reflection. However, there is a balance between getting some relaxation and hiding away. Too much time on your own can get depressing and can lead to you becoming more vulnerable to the voices taking over.

Martin

Martin listens to rock music on his iPod when his voices are troubling him. This helps him to cope as the music drowns out the voices. Martin can also get lost in the music and tune out from what the voices are saying.

Socializing

Socializing is another type of activity that is quite important for coping with voices. Being with other people can keep our minds occupied so that the voices keep out or are quiet. The company of other people can also give us the opportunity to engage in positive activities that can build our self-esteem (we will learn more about the importance of positive self-esteem beliefs in Chapter 6), such as going for a walk, going to the shops or to the cinema or even to the pub (but don't drink too much!). However, voices can sometimes be very disruptive when we are with other people. For example, they can become loud and be very distracting, or say negative things about us or other people in order to spoil the occasion. People who know us and know about our problems will generally cope with this, although it is probably worth explaining to them what's going on, as they may need to give us a little more time to respond to what they say – and sometimes we will just need to be quiet with them. We may want to find specific ways of coping with the voices in social situations. Sometimes going through a relaxation exercise in our minds or focusing on something – possibly what the other person is saying or doing – may help. Sometimes actively daydreaming can help – imagining you are on holiday in a beautiful place, or on a beach, or taking part in an interesting event, e.g. a football match or perhaps acting in a film. However, as already discussed, fighting the voices directly in our minds doesn't usually tend to work.

There are perhaps other social activities you can engage in, such as sports or particular interests that you've enjoyed in the past but that you may have stopped doing because of your voices, or because you lost interest and energy. These might be worth considering again: you might be able to get back into them, with a bit of a push from yourself and others, if they want to help. Doing things together with someone else can often help you rekindle some motivation – if only because you may not want to let down the other person.

There might also be new interests you could try, either on your own or with other people – check the Internet or local libraries for information about clubs and activities that are available in your local area. Online gaming and networking sites can also be a good way of entering a social network, and has the option of staying alone if you feel like it. How you interact with other people depends on the game you choose. These range from very simple shoot-them-up scenarios, which might help you to alleviate frustration, to complex virtual worlds in which you have a valued role to play if you choose it (for example, Second Life). These options are great rehearsals for real-life situations, but be slightly cautious as it is easy to get too absorbed in alternative gaming worlds and forget (or avoid) day-to-day activities such as shopping and cleaning, etc. Also, remember that online gaming and networking may not necessarily help alleviate social isolation.

There are day centres and social groups available for people recovering from hearing distressing voices (or similar problems). These can be very welcoming as they are likely to be accepting and not very demanding in terms of expectations on you to do anything too difficult or stressful. You can speak to your GP or a mental health professional about attending a day centre or joining a social group. Local voluntary services will also have directories of centres and groups, and often post this information on their websites. Although you may feel that you don't want to go somewhere where there are people with mental health problems – either because you think it might be depressing or you don't want to be associated with this group because you don't feel you have the same sort of problems – you won't know until you try.

Martin

Martin uses Facebook to stay in touch with friends that he used to spend time with. He is thinking about asking to meet with some of these old friends, but he feels quite nervous about doing this. He is concerned about how the voices will react. The next step might be to send one of his old friends a text message, or telephone or Skype them. Doing things gradually, in this way, means that Martin can check the friend's response and the response of the voices. If the voices do become troublesome, he may be able to use some of the techniques described in this book in order to manage them and cope with them better – and eventually meet up with a friend.

Work activities offer another way of spending time with other people. Like taking regular exercise, we can begin work activities on our own, if we choose, then gradually build up to work with others. We might begin with household tasks. They may be boring but are often much appreciated. Someone has to tidy the garden, do the shopping, hoover, wash the dishes, do the D-I-Y ... the list is long! These activities can help you in several ways:

1. They provide structure and routine to the day and stop us getting lost in time and voices.

2. They offer an opportunity for us to be appreciated by the other people who will benefit from our efforts – and we all need to feel appreciated, particularly when voices are putting us down.

3. These tasks give us a chance to give to others, which is often underestimated as a source of feeling good about ourselves.

If you're able to venture further afield, work outside the home can be voluntary, paid or involve education – going to college. If you don't feel up to working or don't want to, that's fine – maybe later. However, if you feel up to it, work is a great way of meeting people, keeping occupied and maybe getting some money. Because work involves doing things with other people, it can also be an easier way of socializing and interacting than going out and meeting people in a strictly social setting – when you may feel pressurized to have something to say.

If you don't feel ready for paid work, or there's none around, unpaid voluntary work is often available – again it's worth asking around or looking for information. There is likely to be a Council for Voluntary Service locally, or you could look up

Volunteering England on the Internet. Alternatively, you could just walk into anywhere that uses volunteers – charity shops can be a good starting point, but other places also use volunteers, for example some parks use volunteer gardeners.

Martin

Martin has been doing a lot of the cooking and cleaning at home, which is much appreciated by his family. He is good at it and his confidence has grown after hearing his family give complimentary remarks about his work, thus giving purpose and structure to his day. Boosted by this success, Martin begins to believe a voluntary job might be possible, perhaps leading eventually to paid work.

Mental health care

It may seem strange to think of mental health care as a coping strategy but, for the most part, that's exactly what it is. It is intended to help us be able to cope better. Talking to a mental health worker who understands the experiences that we are having can be hugely beneficial; they may be able to help us work out the best ways of understanding our voices and coping with them – and with other related problems such as anxiety, depression and anger. Some will have particular skills at doing this sort of work, e.g. some clinical psychologists and specially trained nursing or social-work staff. Many staff will have undertaken training to develop their skills, some in Cognitive Behaviour Therapy (see the references at the end of the book for a list of useful resources). You can ask for a referral for therapy from your GP – it is one of the things that all mental health services have to make available. (Mention NICE Guidelines – these are developed by a government agency, the National Institute of Health and Clinical Excellence, to ensure that good-quality treatment is available – see the website address at the end of this book.)

You may be offered therapy and wonder if it really is for you. Even if you do have reservations, it is worth going to the assessment interview and discussing any concerns you have. The voices may tell you not to go, or you may fear that you'll have to talk about things that you don't want to. However, it should be explained to you from the beginning that you will control what is said and the areas to be covered – the therapist may encourage you and support you to deal with difficult issues but it will be in your control. You won't have to say anything you don't want to. You may be doubtful as to whether it is worth the effort or can help. In fact, there is some very good evidence to show that most people do get something useful out of therapy sessions with a properly trained therapist.

And then there is medication. This definitely helps most people with distressing voices in the short term, as it seems to reduce the level of stimulation experienced and the intensity of the voices (even what they say can become less unpleasant – less rude, critical or abusive). Sometimes varying the dose can help – for example, taking an extra tablet when the voices are particularly bad or before an event if you can predict they'll get worse, such as on an important anniversary or before going to meet someone. However, it is very important that you discuss any varying of your medication with your therapist or GP, as it can affect the benefits and side effects that you get from it. It is also very important that you tell them about the benefits attributed to the medication – or any problems that you have with it – so they can adjust the prescription accordingly. For more information about medication, there are many websites, books and leaflets available. See the list of useful organizations at the end of this book.

Exactly how long one should continue taking medication is becoming a hot topic among psychiatric researchers and practitioners. Traditionally, the advice has been that people who have experienced distressing voices need to take medication on a long-term basis – and this is what the government's guidelines say. However, researchers are now beginning to look at what support might help people with distressing voices if they are not taking medication – but it is very early days and we simply don't know at the moment. If you have doubts about taking medication, talk to the person who prescribes it. Stopping it without consulting your doctor or therapist is not a good idea – it inevitably can cause friction with family members or simply cause you uncertainty and anxiety. It is likely to put you at risk of developing a worsening of your voices and other problems. If you have concerns about your medication and don't feel you are being listened to, you might find that a local mental health group, such as MIND or the Hearing Voices Network (see links to websites at the end of this book), can be a source of support. Alternatively, a family member or friend might be able to go with you to see the doctor and help you express your concerns. Don't feel embarrassed about taking someone with you when you go to see your doctor, as it is fairly common practice for physical health problems as well as mental health problems, and it is more important that you feel you have any moral support you need. Some mental health services offer independent advocates who can help you work out what you want to say and support you in doing so. Medication doesn't work for everyone but there are different tablets and injections that you can try – also, switching might help or you could try different doses – but remember it is important to discuss this with your prescriber.

Martin

Martin meets regularly with a mental health worker. He has known this worker for a long time and trusts him enough to talk about his voices. These conversations are helpful as Martin can check the accuracy of some of the things that his voices say.

Martin is prescribed medication for his voices. He takes it most of the time as it helps him to feel less anxious. At first, the tablets helped to control the voices, but the voices don't seem to be affected any more. The tablets sometimes make Martin feel drowsy. When this happens he often misses a dose.

His partner suggests that he discusses this with the psychiatrist who prescribes his medication. Martin and the psychiatrist agree that it would be better for him not to feel drowsy – and so they decide to reduce the dose. The consequence of this is that Martin now takes the medication regularly and this seems to be reducing the distress caused by the voices.

Your ways of coping

Finding successful ways of coping with distressing voices is not always straightforward and so persistence is often the key to finding strategies that work for you. With time, most people find ways of adjusting to the voices and reducing the intensity of distress they can cause. Try using the coping worksheet at the end of this chapter to think about the coping strategies that you use or might want to consider trying out. The worksheet can help you to think about the effectiveness of your coping strategies, and encourage you to try new ways.

Summary

People who hear distressing voices have found many different ways to help them cope with and manage their difficulties. Some are less effective than others, and you may have found some strategies that work well for you. Some of the most effective ways of coping with voices involve trying to manage stress through the use of distraction or relaxation techniques. Other effective techniques involve socializing and spending time with people, which is often a good way to start building positive self-esteem. Mental health services can also help you to cope by providing the opportunity to talk to experts about the voices and by offering medication. There is no one-size-fits-all approach to coping with voices, so it is important to persist until you find a way of coping that works for you.

Key points

- It will help you to cope with voices if you can understand more about them. What do they sound like? Can others hear them? What do they say? Where do they seem to come from? What might have caused them to start?
- Understanding more about your voices can help you to cope better, even if this is difficult to begin with.

- Try a few different coping strategies in order to find some that work for you.
- Keep a record of your different ways of trying to cope and keep monitoring their effectiveness.

Coping worksheet

- What ways do you use now to cope with your voices?

____

____

____

- How effective are they? Can they make the voices worse? Do they work better at particular times, e.g. when you are – or maybe are not – stressed?

____

____

____

- Do you want to try one or a number of new coping strategies? There are three different types to use (see section entitled "Stress management"):

  * What could you do to manage your stress levels? Try to think of one or two things:

  ____

  ____

  ____

* Is there anybody you could see? Any social setting? Try to think of one or two:

____
____
____

* Are there any work activities you could try?

____
____
____

* Is there anything that mental health services could offer – such as treatments or other kinds of help – that you might not have tried in the past?

____
____
____

* Sometimes distractions designed to keep your mind occupied can help, e.g. Sudoku, crosswords, music, listening to the radio, computer games. Can you think of one or two you might try?

____
____
____

- Okay – now is the time to select one new coping strategy and decide when you are going to try it, so which one?

____

____

____

- When are you going to do it?

____

____

____

- When you've tried it, check how effective it was:

  * It may not have solved the problem but did it help just a little?

  * Could you have done it differently?

  * Is it worth using it again? Or trying something different?

  ____

  ____

  ____

Part Three

Changing Beliefs and Relationships

5

Changing beliefs about voices

In Chapter 1 we saw how our thoughts about our voices can influence how we feel. We explained how these thoughts are *beliefs,* not *facts:* they are best guesses about what is happening. Sometimes these beliefs are similar to what the voices say to us. For example, we may believe that the voice is very powerful – and the voices may be telling us that they can make things happen around us. However, sometimes beliefs about our voices are different to what the voices say. For example, Martin and Sarah's voices both said the same thing ('if you go out I will punish you'), but their beliefs were very different. Martin believed that his voices were powerful, had control over him and would cause him harm – resulting in him feeling distressed. Sarah, however, did not believe that her voices were powerful or had any control over her – so she felt irritated rather than distressed by the voice.

The case studies of Martin and Sarah show us that the most important beliefs about voices are usually beliefs about the power of the voice, its intentions towards us and the control the voice has over us. If we believe that the voice is all-powerful (omnipotent), intends to harm us (malevolent) and can control us, this is likely to be distressing. But remember, these beliefs are best guesses. They are not facts. The exercises in this chapter will help you to work out if your beliefs about your voices are good and accurate guesses, or whether they are a bit wide of the mark. Could it be the case that you believe your voices to be more powerful than they actually are?

The beliefs we have about ourselves also have an impact. We saw in Chapter 2 that having negative core beliefs about ourselves can leave us at the mercy of the voices and what they say. While this chapter will focus mainly on changing our beliefs about voices, we also begin to look more closely at our beliefs about ourselves.

What do I think about my voice?

Let's return to the diagram from Chapter 1 that used the ABC model to help us understand the influence of our beliefs. Try filling in the diagram (as shown in Figure 16) to help you think about the beliefs you have about your voices. Before doing this, choose one particular voice to focus on. If you hear only one voice this will be straightforward. If you hear two or more, select the voice that you most want to change. Some people hear lots of voices that are difficult to distinguish from each other – a bit like a crowd. If this is the case for you, choose a belief that you have about the crowd of voices.

Were you able to think about and identify the beliefs you have about your voices? Thinking about our voices in this way may not be easy at first. We don't often think about our thinking! We just think. The questions in Figures 17 and 18 will help us to think about and understand our beliefs about the power and intentions of our voices, and how much control they have over us.

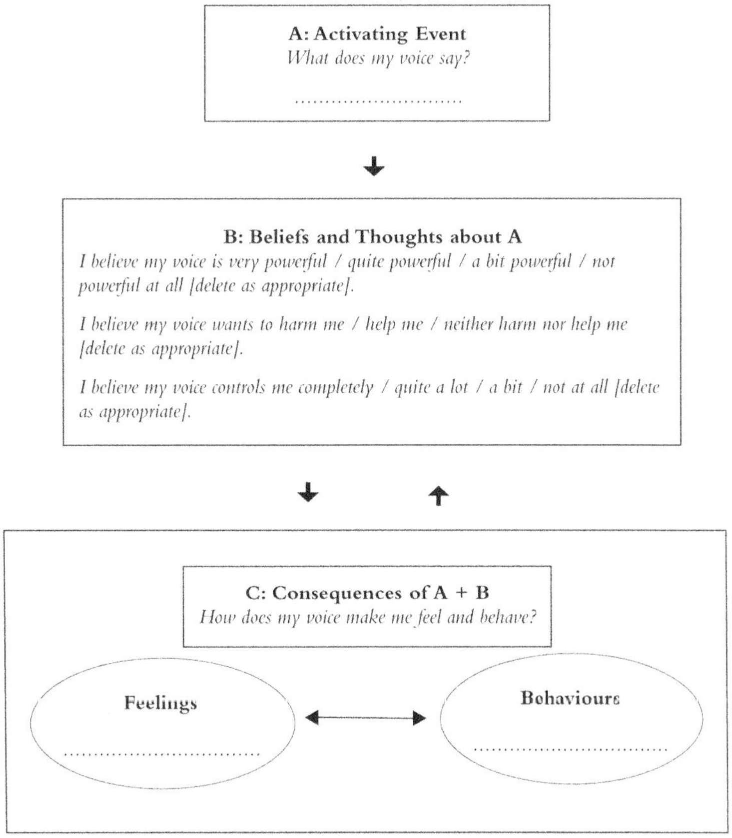

Figure 16: A Cognitive Behaviour Therapy approach to understanding your voices – the ABC model

Figure 17: Rating beliefs about the power and control of my voice (Items taken from the Beliefs About Voices questionnaire – revised, Chadwick et al., 2000)

My voice is very powerful

Disagree (score 0)

Unsure (score 1)

Slightly Agree (score 2)

Strongly Agree (score 3)

My voice seems to know everything about me

Disagree (score 0)

Unsure (score 1)

Slightly Agree (score 2)

Strongly Agree (score 3)

My voice makes me do things I really don't want to do

Disagree (score 0)

Unsure (score 1)

Slightly Agree (score 2)

Strongly Agree (score 3)

I cannot control my voice

Disagree (score 0)

Unsure (score 1)

Slightly Agree (score 2)

Strongly Agree (score 3)

My voice will harm or kill me if I disobey or resist it

Disagree (score 0)

Unsure (score 1)

Slightly Agree (score 2)

Strongly Agree (score 3)

My voice rules my life

Disagree (score 0)

____

____

____

Unsure (score 1)

____

____

____

Slightly Agree (score 2)

____

____

____

Strongly Agree (score 3)

____

____

____

The rating of my belief about my voice's power and control is _____/18

How did you get on? A higher score means a stronger belief in the power and control of the voice, whereas a lower score indicates a belief that the voice has limited power and control. Did your answers give you some clues about your beliefs about the power and control of your voice? Try going back to Figure 16 and review the answers you gave in the B section.

Were your responses accurate or, upon reflection, do they need revising?

Figure 18: Rating beliefs about the harmful intentions of my voice (Items taken from the Beliefs About Voices questionnaire – revised, Chadwick et al., 2000)

My voice is punishing me for something I have done

Disagree (score 0)

____

____

____

Unsure (score 1)

____

____

____

Slightly Agree (score 2)

____

____

____

Strongly Agree (score 3)

____

____

____

My voice is persecuting me for no good reason

Disagree (score 0)

Unsure (score 1)

Slightly Agree (score 2)

Strongly Agree (score 3)

My voice is evil

Disagree (score 0)

Unsure (score 1)

Slightly Agree (score 2)

Strongly Agree (score 3)

My voice want to harm me

Disagree (score 0)

Unsure (score 1)

Slightly Agree (score 2)

Strongly Agree (score 3)

My voice wants me to do bad things

Disagree (score 0)

Unsure (score 1)

Slightly Agree (score 2)

Strongly Agree (score 3)

My voice is trying to corrupt or destroy me

Disagree (score 0)

____
____
____

Unsure (score 1)

____
____
____

Slightly Agree (score 2)

____
____
____

Strongly Agree (score 3)

____
____
____

The rating of my belief about my voice's harmful intentions is __/18

How did you get on? Did your answers give you some clues about your beliefs about the harmful intentions of your voice? Try going back to Figure 16 and change or add to the answers you gave in the B section. Martin's beliefs about his voices are written below.

Martin

*I believe my voice is **very powerful** quite powerful/a bit powerful/not powerful at all*

*I believe my voice wants to **harm me** /help me/neither harm nor help me*

*I believe my voice controls me **completely** /quite a lot/a bit/not at all*

Step 1 – naming beliefs about voices

The first step in assessing the accuracy of your beliefs about your voices is to select one belief to work on. Try looking at the beliefs about your voice's power, control and intentions that you rated in Figures 17 and 18 and choose one highly rated belief (score of 2 or 3) to start working on. To start with it might be helpful to choose a belief that is not too strong or painful to think about. When you feel more confident in how to question beliefs about your voices, you can repeat this process with other, more strongly held beliefs.

Once you have chosen a belief to start working on you may want to write down the belief:

> Belief about voice to work on: 'I believe my voice is _____'

Martin

Let's return to thinking about Martin. Earlier in this chapter we looked at Martin's beliefs that he developed about his voices. These beliefs make sense when we think about the difficulties that Martin has experienced during his life – his stepfather was powerful, harmed Martin and his mother, and had control over them. For this exercise Martin has chosen to work on his belief about the power of his voice.

Belief about voice to work on: 'I believe my voice is very powerful'

Step 2 – rating how much we believe the beliefs about our voices

Now we have chosen a belief to work on, the next step is to decide how much we believe this belief is true. Below you might want to write down how much you believe your chosen belief about your voice is true. At the moment you might believe it is true with absolute certainty, in which case you might say you are 100 per cent certain it is true. You might decide that you are unsure if it is true and that you are only about 50 per cent certain.

Right now I believe this belief about my voice is true with about ______ per cent certainty.

Martin

Right now I think that my belief that my voice is very powerful is true with about ***100*** per cent certainty.

Step 3 – noticing the impact of the beliefs about voices

When you look at the belief about your voice that you have chosen, how do you feel? In the space below you can write down how you feel when you think about the belief, and how this affects your behaviour and bodily sensations. If you notice different feelings, then you can use a separate row to write about each one.

When I think about this belief about my voice:

I feel

(Name the feeling in one word)

____

____

____

Strength of feeling

(Where 100% means the feeling is as strong as possible)

Feelings in body

(Do you notice anything in your body when you feel this way?)

I feel

(Name the feeling in one word)

Strength of feeling

(Where 100% means the feeling is as strong as possible)

Feelings in body

(Do you notice anything in your body when you feel this way?)

I feel

(Name the feeling in one word)

Strength of feeling

(Where 100% means the feeling is as strong as possible)

Feelings in body

(Do you notice anything in your body when you feel this way?)

I feel

Strength of feeling

(Where 100% means the feeling is as strong as possible)

____

____

____

Feelings in body

(Do you notice anything in your body when you feel this way?)

____

____

____

It is important to notice these feelings and bodily sensations, because they can unhelpfully act as evidence that the belief about our voice is true. So, if we feel intimidated and notice our heart racing, we might conclude that this is because our voice is very powerful. Yet, it is the belief that the voice is powerful that makes us feel intimidated, rather than the actual power of the voice. And as we have previously seen, this belief is just a best guess.

Martin

When I think about the belief that my voice is very powerful:

I feel

(Name the feeling in one word)

Strength of feeling

(Where 100% means the feeling is as strong as possible)

Feelings in body

(Do you notice anything in your body when you feel this way?)

I feel

Intimidated

Strength of feeling

80%

Feelings in body

Heart beating quickly, tense

I feel

Angry

Strength of feeling

100%

Feelings in body

Like I'm going to burst

Our beliefs, feelings and bodily sensations are closely linked – as we saw in the ABC model. If we review the evidence and conclude that our voice is less powerful, this will weaken the strength of our feelings and bodily sensations. These weakened feelings and bodily sensations will then be less likely to offer evidence that supports our belief that the voice is very powerful; thus our belief will diminish. So, reviewing the evidence that supports the belief about your voice is very important because it can have the positive effect of undermining your belief.

Step 4 – exploring the evidence

Cognitive Behaviour Therapy is not about positive thinking, it is about carefully and accurately looking at *evidence.* In this fourth step, we ask ourselves is there any *evidence* or experiences that do not fit with our belief about the voice? Is there any *evidence* or experiences that mean that our belief about our voice is not, in fact, completely true?

Exercise:

Let's continue to work on the belief about your voice that you chose in Step 1. Now, using Table 2, write down any evidence or experiences that mean that the belief you have chosen is not completely true all of the time. Some examples are provided to get you started.

Table 2: Reviewing the evidence

Belief about voice: *'I believe my voice is very powerful _____'*

Evidence and experiences that mean this belief about my voice is ***not*** completely true all of the time:

1. *I didn't harm myself when my voice told me to do this and nothing bad happened*
2. *My voice has never actually harmed me*
3. *I enjoyed spending time with my friend even though my voice was trying to ruin it by threatening me and shouting*
4. *I was able to concentrate on reading a book despite my voice talking and trying to distract me*
5. *Just briefly, I felt good about myself after I finished reading, even though my voice was saying that I was useless and could only read a few pages*
6.
7.
8.
9.
10.

If you had a go at filling in Table 2, how did you find it? Was it easy to do or difficult? Most people find it difficult at first to notice evidence or experiences that do not fit with the beliefs they hold about their voices. Remember from Chapter 2 that the human mind works by searching for evidence that our beliefs are true, and tends to ignore evidence that does not fit with our beliefs. This means that noticing and writing down evidence that does not fit with our beliefs about our voices is making our mind do something it does not naturally want to do!

Don't worry if you found this exercise difficult. Doing the following might help you:

- Look back over the entire time that you have heard the voices. Can you find any evidence or experiences that do not fit with the belief you have chosen to work on?

- Are you giving yourself enough chances to gather evidence that will help you to challenge the belief you hold about your voices? Perhaps you are avoiding spending time with people or avoiding going out because you're worried that the belief about your voices might be true. In this case, you might want to plan activities you can do that might help you to gather evidence to add to the list. For example, if you believe that your voices are very powerful, you could try to do something that your voices usually try to prevent you from doing. In Table 2, reading a book was an activity that provided some evidence that the voice could not necessarily prevent something from happening. It is best to start with a straightforward activity – such as reading – that does not feel too challenging.

Most people will take a long time to add evidence and experiences to the list. This is because thinking in this way about your voices and yourself can feel very different to how you usually think about them. It may also feel a bit risky to think in ways that your voices may disapprove of. Your voices may even tell you not to do this. This is a common response from voices when a client starts a course of CBT with us. The voices try to sabotage the attempts of the client to change their experience of hearing voices. We encourage clients to take one step at a time, taking the opportunity to review the evidence as each step is taken. For example, if your voices told you not to add anything to the list and you were able to do this anyway, how did your voices respond? What you learn about your voices in this instance may form the next valuable piece of evidence. This gradual, step-by-step process may mean that the list takes a few weeks to complete. This might mean that you will want to come back to the list every week or so, until you have completed it.

Martin

Belief about voice: *'I believe my voice is very powerful'* _____

Evidence and experiences that mean this belief about my voice is ***not*** completely true all of the time:

1. *Occasionally I have not obeyed the voice and nothing terrible has happened*

2. *My voice has never actually carried out any of its threats*

3. *I went out yesterday and nothing bad happened to me*

Step 5 – how much do I believe the beliefs about the voices now?

When you have completed Step 4 (remembering that this may take a few weeks) you might want to ask yourself again how much you believe your chosen belief is true. Before you do this, spend a few moments reading through the evidence you have gathered.

After looking at the evidence, complete the sentence below:

> I believe the belief about my voice is true with about ______ per cent certainty.

How does this rating compare with the rating you gave in Step 2? You might notice that you believe the belief with less certainty now that you have had a chance to gather new evidence that contradicts your old beliefs. On the other hand, you might notice that you believe it just as strongly as you did in Step 2. This is not unusual because, as we now know, our beliefs about our voices have often been around for a long time and they can be difficult to change. If this happens, you may benefit from going back to Step 4 and identifying new experiences and evidence that you can gather that will demonstrate that what your voice says is not completely true all of the time. Alternatively, you might want to go to Chapter 6 and start to think in more depth about the beliefs you have about yourself. If you can develop more positive beliefs about yourself, then this will help you to think differently about your voices.

Starting to change beliefs about yourself

How did you find the exercises in Steps 1 to 5? Were you able to name a belief about your voice, rate how much you believed it, think about the impact of this belief, explore evidence for its accuracy and re-rate it? Did anything change? This work can be very difficult, and may not be immediately helpful for everyone. An alternative approach is to think about your beliefs about yourself, rather than your voice. We will do lots of this in Chapter 6 when we look at how to change the negative core beliefs we often have about ourselves. As a warm-up, try working through

Steps 2, 3, 4 and 5 again but this time examining the following belief:

> Belief about self to work on: *'I believe I have personal control, even when my voice is active.'*

You can use Step 2 to rate how much you believe this belief; Step 3 to consider the impact of holding this belief; Step 4 to explore the evidence that supports this belief; and Step 5 to revisit how much you believe the belief in the light of the evidence.

Next steps

This chapter has mainly focused on trying to change your beliefs about your voices. If you have managed to change the way you see your voices – and things are now better for you – this is really good news. You may want to continue working on other beliefs about your voices in order to maintain these changes and maybe make further changes. Or you might want to try to change beliefs about other voices that you hear. Additionally, you may want to build on the changes in your beliefs about the voices by thinking more about how you see yourself, and how to change beliefs about yourself for the better. Chapter 6 will help you do this.

If, on the other hand, it may have been too difficult for you to change your beliefs about your voices at the moment, don't worry: Chapter 6 can offer a different and possibly more positive approach for you.

There is no right place to start when you are trying to change the way things are with your voices. Just do what you feel comfortable doing.

Martin

Belief about self to work on: 'I believe I have personal control, even when the voice is active'

Right now I think that my belief about personal control is true with about ***30*** per cent certainty.

When I think about my belief about personal control:

I feel

(Name the feeling in one word)

A bit stronger

Strength of feeling

(Where 100% means the feeling is as strong as possible)

30%

Feelings in body

(Do you notice anything in your body when you feel this way?)

A bit calmer

I feel

(Name the feeling in one word)

Hopeful

Strength of feeling

(Where 100% means the feeling is as strong as possible)

40%

Feelings in body

(Do you notice anything in your body when you feel this way?)

Lighter

Belief about voice: *'I believe I have personal control, even when my voice is active'*

Evidence and experiences that support this belief:

1. *I went out yesterday, even though the voices were telling me not to*

2. *I was able to have a conversation with mum, even when the voices were talking*

3. *I have started to re-connect with old friends*

After looking at the evidence, I believe my belief about personal control is true with about *50 per cent* certainty

Summary

It is common for us to believe that voices are all-powerful, have control over us and want to harm us. If we believe these things about our voices then we are likely to feel distressed a lot of the time. We can start to overcome this distress by assessing the accuracy of these beliefs. Once we start to do this, we may find that there is a lot of evidence that these beliefs are not true all of the time. As we begin to challenge our beliefs about our voices, we may start to notice that the voices lose some of their power and control over us, and we start to feel more in charge of our lives.

Key points

- If we believe our voices have power and control over us, and want to harm us, this can be very distressing.
- However, beliefs are not facts; they are best guesses and can sometimes be wide of the mark.
- We can begin to overcome the distress caused by our voices by naming our beliefs about them and learning about how these beliefs affect us.
- When we are familiar with these beliefs and their effects, we can challenge the accuracy of our beliefs about our voices.

- We can challenge the accuracy of our beliefs about our voices by gathering evidence that suggests that our beliefs are not true all of the time.
- After weighing up the evidence, we might conclude that our voices are maybe less powerful than we previously thought, and maybe we have more control than we thought.
- Challenging our beliefs about our voices can be difficult. An alternative approach is to gather evidence in support of a positive belief about our personal control.
- Challenging our beliefs about our voices is one way to overcome our distressing voices. Another approach is to challenge the beliefs we hold about ourselves. We will look at this in more detail in the next chapter.

6

Overcoming low self-esteem and distressing voices

In Chapter 2, we saw that being distressed by hearing voices usually goes hand in hand with low self-esteem. That is, people who feel distressed when hearing voices often have a low opinion of themselves. They may believe deep down that they are no good, not worth loving, or are incapable. In Cognitive Behaviour Therapy we call these kinds of beliefs about ourselves 'negative core beliefs'.

We also saw in Chapter 2 that negative core beliefs about ourselves usually start in early childhood and are our way of making sense of our life experiences. So, as young children we might decide that we are 'no good' because we are being bullied at school. The simple fact is that people who are distressed by hearing voices are much more likely than other people to have had difficult childhood experiences. So it is not surprising to learn that people who are distressed by voices often have negative core beliefs about themselves.

Once we have developed a negative core belief (such as 'I'm no good') our minds look for reasons why it is true and ignore the reasons why it might not be true. This means that negative beliefs about ourselves can become stronger as we get older. The important thing to remember about negative core beliefs is that, in fact, they are rarely true.

In this chapter, we look at ways of overcoming low self-esteem. A lot of the ideas put forward are about overcoming low self-esteem in general, rather than specifically in relation to hearing voices. After all, low self-esteem can affect us all.

Before we start, we need to remember that our negative core beliefs have usually been around since we were young children. This can mean that they are difficult to change. So, as well as looking at ways of changing negative core beliefs, we also look at ways of building up our self-esteem by strengthening positive beliefs about ourselves.

Low self-esteem and negative core beliefs

Do I have low self-esteem?

In Chapter 2 we suggested some questions that you could ask yourself to find out if you have problems with low self-esteem. Here are the questions again – take a few minutes to read through and answer them again, making a note of your answers on a piece of paper. The higher the score, the higher your self-esteem (the maximum possible score is 30) and most people score 17 or more on the questionnaire.

From your answers, do you think you might have low self-esteem? If you do, then you might find the ideas in this chapter helpful.

Figure 19: Rating your self-esteem (Rosenberg Self-Esteem Scale, Rosenberg 1965)

1. On the whole I am satisfied with myself.

Strongly Agree

3

Agree

2

Disagree

1

Strongly Disagree

0

2. At times, I think I am no good at all.

Strongly Agree

0

Agree

1

Disagree

2

Strongly Disagree

3

3. I feel that I have a number of good qualities.

Strongly Agree

3

Agree

2

Disagree

1

Strongly Disagree

0

4. I am able to do things as well as most other people.

Strongly Agree

3

Agree

2

Disagree

1

Strongly Disagree

0

5. I feel I do not have much to be proud of.

Strongly Agree

0

Agree

1

Disagree

2

Strongly Disagree

3

6. I certainly feel useless at times.

Strongly Agree

0

Agree

1

Disagree

2

3

7. I feel that I'm a person of worth, at least on an equal plane with others.

Strongly Agree

3

Agree

2

Disagree

1

Strongly Disagree

0

8. I wish I could have more respect for myself.

Strongly Agree

0

Agree

1

Disagree

2

Strongly Disagree

3

9. All in all, I am inclined to feel that I am a failure.

Strongly Agree

0

Agree

1

Disagree

2

Strongly Disagree

3

10. I take a positive attitude towards myself.

Strongly Agree

3

Agree

2

Disagree

1

Strongly Disagree

0

Total score=______/30

Do I have negative core beliefs about myself?

We saw earlier that core beliefs are the way we think about ourselves deep down. These are beliefs that have often been around since we were young children. Negative core beliefs lie at the heart of low self-esteem. We can identify our core beliefs as 'I am...' statements. For example, 'I am kind', 'I am lazy', 'I am conscientious'. Once we can identify our negative core beliefs it is easier to start to question how accurate they really are.

Do any of the negative core belief statements below *seem* true about you? Some of these statements might seem true all or most of the time, or they might just seem true some of the time. Take a few moments to read through these statements and ask yourself if, at least sometimes, you believe these things are true.

- I am not okay as I am.
- I am no good at all.
- I don't have any good qualities.
- I am useless.
- I am not worthwhile.
- I am a failure.
- I am weak.

- I am vulnerable.
- I am bad.

At this point, it is important to note that a lot of people will believe at least some of these statements some of the time. In particular, we know that people who are distressed by hearing voices are more likely than other people to believe negative things about themselves. As we have learnt, although these things can *seem* true about ourselves, they are almost certainly not true.

Questioning our negative core beliefs

On the next few pages you will find a step-by-step approach to questioning the accuracy of negative core beliefs. Remember that because negative core beliefs have been around a long time they are often deeply rooted in our minds. This means that we will probably not be able to get rid of them altogether. In this section, we will look at ways of questioning them: once we can question how accurate our core beliefs are they can have less of an emotional impact.

Step 1: Naming negative core beliefs

The first step in overcoming low self-esteem is to recognize and name your negative core beliefs. Looking at the negative statements listed opposite, choose one belief to start working on (or you might want to choose a different 'I am...' belief that is not in the list). To start with, it might be helpful to choose a core belief that is not too strong or painful to think about. Then, when you feel more confident in how to question your negative core beliefs, you can repeat this process with other, more strongly held beliefs.

Once you have chosen a core belief to start working on, write it down below, or on a piece of paper or in a notebook:

Negative core belief: 'I am _____'

Martin

Let's return to thinking about Martin. In Chapter 2 we looked at Martin's negative core beliefs that he developed, for good reasons, in response to some very difficult early life experiences. Martin came to the conclusion that he was weak and vulnerable, no good and not worth anything. For this exercise, Martin has chosen to work on his belief that he is weak and vulnerable.

Negative core belief to work on:

'I am ***weak and vulnerable'***

Step 2: Rating how much we believe negative core beliefs

Now that you have chosen a belief to work on, the next step is to decide how much you believe this negative core belief is true. Below you might want to write down how much you believe your chosen core belief is true about you. At the moment, you might believe it is true with absolute certainty, in which case you might say you are 100 per cent certain it is true. Or you might decide that you are unsure if it is completely true and that you are only about 50 per cent certain.

> Right now I believe this core belief is true with about ______ per cent certainty.

Martin
Right now I believe this core belief is true with about ***90*** per cent certainty.

Step 3: Noticing the impact of your negative core belief

When you look at the core belief you have chosen, how does it make you feel and how strong are these feelings? In the space below, or in your notebook, write down how you feel when the negative core belief is around. Make a note of the bodily sensations that you notice in response to the belief and how strong these feelings are. If you notice different feelings you can use a separate row to write about each one.

I feel (Name the feeling in one word)

Strength of feeling (%) (Where 100% means the feeling is as strong as possible)

Feelings in body (Do you notice anything in your body when you feel this way?)

I feel (Name the feeling in one word)

Strength of feeling (%) (Where 100% means the feeling is as strong as possible)

Feelings in body (Do you notice anything in your body when you feel this way?)

I feel (Name the feeling in one word)

Strength of feeling (%) (Where 100% means the feeling is as strong as possible)

Feelings in body (Do you notice anything in your body when you feel this way?)

Martin's completed example is given below:

Martin

When I think about this negative core belief:

I feel (Name the feeling in one word)

Frightened

Strength of feeling % (Where 100% means the feeling is as strong as possible)

70%

Feelings in body (Do you notice anything in your body when you feel this way?)

Heart beating fast, headache

I feel (Name the feeling in one word)

Down

Strength of feeling % (Where 100% means the feeling is as strong as possible)

80%

Feelings in body (Do you notice anything in your body when you feel this way?)

No energy, tired all the time

Step 4: Exploring the evidence

Cognitive Behaviour Therapy is not about positive thinking, it is about carefully and accurately looking at *evidence.* In this fourth step, we ask ourselves is there any evidence or have we had any experiences that do not fit with our negative core belief? Is there any evidence or have we had any experiences that mean that our negative core belief is not completely true?

In the space below, or in your notebook, write down any evidence or experiences that mean that the negative core belief you have chosen to focus on is not completely true all of the time.

> Negative Core Belief: 'I am_____'
>
> Evidence and experiences that mean this negative core belief is not completely true all of the time.
>
> 1.
> 2.
> 3.
> 4.
> 5.
> 6.
> 7.
> 8.
> 9.
> 10.

If you had a go at adding evidence or experiences to the list how did you find it? Was it easy to do or difficult? Most people find it difficult at first to notice evidence or experiences that do not fit with their deeply held negative core beliefs. Remember from Chapter 2 that the human mind works by searching for evidence that our beliefs *are* true and ignores evidence that does not fit with our beliefs. This means that noticing and writing down evidence that does not fit with our beliefs can be very challenging and difficult at first.

If you found this exercise difficult, the following might help:

- If there is anyone you trust, ask them to suggest evidence or experiences to add to the list. You may find it difficult to believe what the other person says – you may notice thoughts popping into your mind such as 'they are only saying that to be nice'. If this happens, see if you can keep an open mind. Ask yourself whether or not the suggestion is good evidence to add to the list.
- Look back over the whole of your life for evidence or experiences that do not fit with the negative core belief you have chosen to work on. Is there any evidence from when you were a baby or toddler? From when you were a young child, older child or teenager? From when you were a young adult, and so on?
- Are you giving yourself enough chances to gather evidence that will help you to challenge your negative core belief? Perhaps you are avoiding spending time with people or going out because you are worried that the core belief might be true. In this case you might want to plan activities you

can do that might help you to gather evidence to add to the list.

Most people will take a long time to add evidence and experiences to the list; it can take a few weeks or longer to complete. This might mean that you will want to come back to the list every week or so, until you have completed it.

Martin

Negative Core Belief: *'I am **weak and vulnerable'***

Evidence and experiences that mean this negative core belief is not completely true all of the time.

1. *I live on my own and manage without help from anyone*

2. *I joined the army and completed the training, some people had to drop out*

3. *I am physically quite strong*

Step 5: How much do I believe the negative core belief now?

When you have completed the list in Step 4 (remembering that this may take a few weeks), you might want to ask yourself again how much you believe your chosen negative core belief is true. Before you do this, spend a few moments reading through the evidence you have gathered.

After looking at the evidence:

> I believe the negative core belief is true with about ______ per cent certainty.

How does this rating compare with the rating you gave in Step 2? You might notice that you believe the negative core belief with less certainty now that you have had a chance to gather and assess the evidence. On the other hand, you might notice that you believe it as strongly as you did in Step 2. This is not unusual, because as we now know, negative core beliefs have been around in our lives for a long time and they are difficult to change. This is why it can be a good idea to spend a few weeks or longer gathering evidence that does not support our negative core beliefs. In the next section we look at ways of identifying and strengthening alternative, more positive beliefs about ourselves.

Alternative beliefs

If we experience low self-esteem we might find that we dwell on the negative thoughts and feelings that come with negative core beliefs. This can leave us little time to notice how we really are – we can spend so much time dwelling on negative thoughts and feelings about ourselves that we fail to notice our positive qualities. Once again, this is particularly true for people who are distressed by hearing voices. People who feel distressed in response to hearing voices are less likely than other people to think positive things about themselves.

We know it is difficult to change deep-rooted negative core beliefs – we might be able to change how much we believe they are true, but they may not go away for good. This is not because they are true, but simply because they have become strongly rooted in our minds. In this section, we look at ways of identifying and strengthening alternative, more positive beliefs about ourselves. This can be particularly helpful for people distressed by hearing voices, who may have very few and very weakly held positive beliefs about themselves.

The steps outlined in the next few pages are similar to the steps we followed in identifying and assessing negative core beliefs. This time we will undertake a similar set of steps in order to identify and strengthen *positive* core beliefs. Once again, this is not about 'positive thinking' but about carefully and accurately noticing evidence and experiences that support a positive view of ourselves.

Step 1: Identify an alternative belief about ourselves

As in the previous section, we start with identifying one alternative, more positive belief about ourselves.

We can repeat this process with other beliefs, but it is helpful to start by focusing on one belief that we want to work on.

There are a number of ways in which we can identify an alternative belief. Choose the one that makes most sense to you:

- Look at the evidence you wrote down in Step 4 in the previous section. Take your time to carefully read through the evidence. Imagine you are reading it about someone else – maybe someone you care about. What conclusion do you come to about this person? Can you write this as an 'I am...' statement:

  Alternative belief: 'I am ______'

- Take a moment to remember a recent time when you felt okay about yourself as a person. This might have only lasted a few moments but, as best you can, see if you can remember a recent occasion when you had this feeling. If you can't think of a recent time when this has happened then, as best you can, remember a time in your past when you felt okay about yourself.

  If you can remember a time when you felt okay about yourself, try to remember the situation as clearly as possible (it might help to close your eyes to do this). Take a few moments to remember where you were, and what you could see, hear, smell, taste and feel.

When you have done this, bring to mind how you were feeling at the time, any sensations in your body and thoughts that were going through your mind.

Now try to remember how you saw yourself as a person in that moment. Can you write this as an 'I am...' statement?

Alternative belief: 'I am _____'

- If none of these ways of identifying an alternative core belief make sense for you, look at some possible alternative beliefs in the list below – and perhaps you might want to choose one that you can identify with already, even if only slightly:

  * I am worthy of respect.

  * I am valuable.

  * I am talented.

  * I am successful.

  * I am good.

  * I am interesting.

Alternative belief to work on: 'I am _____'

Martin

Alternative self-esteem belief to work on: *'I am **likeable'.***

Step 2: How much do I believe this alternative belief?

How much do you believe this alternative belief is true? You may not believe it at all, or you may only believe it is true with about 10 per cent certainty. On the other hand, you may be pretty sure that it is true. Write down how much you believe it is true right now.

Right now I believe this is true with about ______ per cent certainty.

Martin

Right now I believe this is true with about ***20*** per cent certainty.

Step 3: Looking at the evidence

Using the space below, write down evidence or experiences that support your alternative belief. This could be any evidence or experiences that suggest your alternative belief is true. This will include experiences you have had recently, as well as experiences from different times in your life.

Negative Core Belief: 'I am_____'
Evidence and experiences that support this belief:
1.
2.
3.
4.
5.
6.
7.
8.
9.
10.

Just as with noticing evidence that challenges our negative core beliefs, we can find it difficult to notice evidence and experiences that support a more positive view of ourselves. If you find this exercise difficult, try asking someone you trust to suggest evidence or experiences to add to the list. You might prefer to imagine what someone you trust or care about would suggest as evidence. Remember that adding evidence to the list might take a few weeks or more, as our minds might be used to ignoring evidence or experiences that fit with a more positive view of ourselves.

Martin

Alternative self-esteem belief: *'I am **likeable**'*

Evidence and experiences that support this belief:

1. *Pete keeps coming around, I guess he wouldn't if he didn't like me*

2. *I treat people pretty well and try not to offend anyone*

3. *A woman in the shop is always really friendly to me and asks how I am*

Step 4: Putting our alternative belief into practice

Have another look at the alternative belief you have identified. What would you be *doing* differently if you believed it was true with a little more certainty?

Use the space below to write down the kinds of things you might be doing differently if you really believed your new, alternative belief was true. What would you be doing that you are not doing now?

Alternative belief: 'I am _____'

If I believed this was true with 100 per cent certainty I would be doing:

1. ______
2. ______
3. ______
4. ______
5. ______

Step 4 is about starting to act *as if* your new, alternative belief is true, even when you don't believe it is true. This might seem like an odd thing to do. We might think we have to wait until we believe it is true before changing our behaviour. The problem with this is that often we behave in ways that fit with our negative core beliefs. What might happen if we started to behave in ways that fitted with our new, more positive beliefs about ourselves?

Of course, this isn't easy to do. There might be lots of thoughts popping into your mind right now that give you reasons not to act as if your alternative belief is true – 'it won't work out', 'you'll only prove it isn't true'. These thoughts might come from our negative core beliefs.

If acting *as if* your alternative belief is true seems scary, then you might prefer at first to start to make small changes in the right direction. Maybe you can ask yourself if there is one thing you could do that fits with your new, more positive belief.

You can think of this as 'testing out' your new, alternative belief. What happens when you act as if your new belief is true? Have you noticed any new evidence or experiences that you could add to your list in section entitled "Step 3: Looking at the evidence"

Martin

Alternative self-esteem belief: *'I am **likeable**'.*

If I believed this was true with 100 per cent certainty I would be doing:

1. *Calling Pete and saying about meeting up, not just waiting for him to come around all the time*

2. *Trying to find more of my old friends on facebook and getting back in touch*

3. *Smiling at people more (in shops and other places)*

In the example above you can see the things that Martin decided to do that fitted with his new belief. Of all the people he knew, Martin trusted his friend Pete the most. However, he realized that he always waited for Pete to come round, Martin never contacted him. He realized that this pattern might never change unless he took the step of doing things differently, and so he decided that he would call Pete and suggest meeting up. Martin felt anxious before calling Pete, his heart was beating fast and he had a knot in his stomach. He kept thinking that Pete would say no. However, he was able to remind himself of the evidence he had written down – that he was likeable – and he was able to pick up the phone and call his friend. To his surprise and relief, Pete seemed genuinely happy to hear from him and immediately agreed to meeting up that evening. Martin then added this as evidence to his list of reasons to support his new belief.

Following this experience, Martin started to call Pete about once a week to suggest meeting up, rather than always waiting for Pete to call round. This led Martin to make contact through Facebook with some of his old friends he had lost touch with. Some of them didn't reply but one of his old friends, Duncan, got back in touch and they started meeting up every now and then to play pool in a local pub.

One of the reasons that Martin wasn't too sure that he was likeable was that people didn't usually smile at him in shops or in other places. However, after his positive experiences with Pete and Duncan, he realized that he never smiled at other people either, and so Martin decided to smile at people more often. When he did this, he noticed that people usually smiled back and even occasionally started making conversation with him. This was more evidence for Martin to add to the list to support his new belief, and was another good example of how acting as if our new beliefs are true (even when we don't believe them) can help to strengthen these beliefs.

We can see that Martin started with Step 4 by choosing a relatively easy thing to do – he trusted Pete more than anyone. Once this turned out okay, Martin was able to choose a slightly more challenging task of contacting old friends, and when this worked out well he was able to take the next step of smiling at people he didn't know.

Step 5: How much do I believe my new belief now?

Once you have spent time gathering evidence that your new belief is true, and once you have had the chance to practise acting as if it is true, you might want to think about how much you believe your new belief. You can use the space below to rate how certain you are that your alternative belief is true.

Alternative belief: ______

Right now I believe this is true with about ______ per cent certainty.

If you have found this helpful, you might want to look again at some of the other alternative beliefs you noted in Step 1 and repeat the five steps.

Martin

Alternative self-esteem belief: *'I am **likeable**'.*

Right now I believe this is true with about: ***60*** per cent certainty.

Acceptance

So far in this chapter we have looked at ways of assessing negative core beliefs about ourselves and at ways of noticing and strengthening alternative, more positive beliefs. As we now know, however, core beliefs about ourselves are usually deeply rooted in our minds and, because of this, they can sometimes be difficult to change.

What do we mean by acceptance?

Negative core beliefs can give rise to a stream of negative thoughts about ourselves. Stop for a moment and notice if there are any negative, self-critical thoughts running through your mind. These negative thoughts pop into our minds automatically and are often outside of our awareness. This is quite a common experience for lots of people but it seems to be especially common for people who are distressed by hearing voices.

If our negative core beliefs have been around for a long time, we might find that these self-critical thoughts pop into our minds a lot of the time. Acceptance means learning to accept that this is how our minds work – accepting that we cannot control the thoughts that pop into our minds. At the same time, acceptance also means learning that what our minds say – the negative thoughts that pop into our minds – are often not true. We remind ourselves that *thoughts are just thoughts, they are not facts.*

The same applies to hearing voices. We will often find that we cannot stop the voices from speaking. Acceptance of voices means the same as acceptance of negative thoughts. In other words, we can learn to accept that the voices are there – and that we may not be able to stop them – but we can learn to respond to them in a different way.

Acceptance means learning not to believe what the voices say and reminding ourselves that the things voices say are often not true. When the voices make unpleasant comments, we can remind ourselves that *voices do not always speak the truth.*

Learning to accept difficult experiences is not easy. However, here are three steps that we might find helpful:

Step 1: Stop and notice negative thoughts and voice comments

Stop and notice negative thoughts popping into your mind. Pause for a moment and notice negative voice comments.

- How do you feel when these thoughts or voices come into your mind?
- What do you notice in your body?

Step 2: Remind yourself that thoughts and voice comments are not facts

Look at the evidence you have written down in Table 2. Remind yourself that negative thoughts and voice comments may *feel* true but this does not mean they are true. See if you can allow negative thoughts and voice comments into your mind and then let them go, without getting drawn into thinking about them or worrying about them.

Step 3: Notice positive experiences

Practise bringing awareness to your new positive beliefs and experiences. Even if these experiences do not happen very often, try as best you can to really notice what it is like when you feel okay about yourself. See if you can remember a recent time when you felt okay about yourself:

- How did you feel?
- What was happening in your body?
- What thoughts were going through your mind?
- What happened to your voices?

- If the voices were still there was it easier to let them pass by without getting drawn into them?

Martin and acceptance

Martin practised these three steps and, in Step 1, he was surprised to notice how often his mind contained negative thoughts and voice comments. When these negative thoughts and voices were around, Martin noticed unpleasant feelings in his body. In particular, he noticed a tight knot in his stomach. In Step 2, Martin was then able to remind himself that the negative thoughts and voice comments were not necessarily true. He told himself 'it is just a thought' and 'it is just a voice comment'. Finally, in Step 3 Martin was able to remember a recent time when he felt okay about himself. This was when he had been out for a coffee with his friend Pete – and Pete had told him what a good time he'd had and that they should go out more often. Martin remembered feeling happy and pleased, and the usual tension in his body lifting, so that his body felt light and relaxed. The usual negative thoughts and voices did not seem to be there for a few hours after meeting Pete and, when they did come into his mind, he was better able than usual to just let them go without getting drawn into them.

Martin overcoming low self-esteem

We saw in Chapter 2 that Martin had negative core beliefs: that he was no good and that he was weak and vulnerable. This made it very easy for him to believe the voices when they made unpleasant and abusive remarks about him. After following the steps set out in this chapter, he found that he didn't believe his negative core beliefs as strongly any more, and that he had uncovered some positive beliefs about himself, such as 'I am likeable' and 'I am capable'. Although the voices might still make unpleasant comments about him, Martin began practising acceptance and noticed that he didn't believe the voices' comments as much as he used to. So, when the voices told him that no one likes him, he was able to notice this comment and then remind himself that this is not true. As a result, although the voices were still around and still made unpleasant comments, Martin did not feel as distressed by the voices as he used to. He had begun to go out more with his friends Pete and Duncan, and began to consider looking for voluntary work, and maybe some paid work at some point in the future, all of which might provide evidence to support his new, positive beliefs about himself.

Summary

It is common to have low self-esteem if we are distressed by hearing voices. If we have low self-esteem it is easier for us to believe unpleasant or frightening voice comments. Negative core beliefs about ourselves (negative 'I am...' statements) are at the heart of low self-esteem and we can start to overcome low self-esteem by assessing the accuracy of these beliefs. Once we start to do this, we may find that there is a lot of evidence that these beliefs are not, in fact, true. In addition to questioning the accuracy of our negative core beliefs, we can also identify positive beliefs about ourselves and work to make these stronger. As we begin to overcome low self-esteem, we may start to notice that the voices lose some of their power and control over us, and we start to feel more in charge of our lives.

Key points

- If we believe negative things about ourselves then it is easier to believe that the voices we hear have power and control over us and that any unpleasant comments they make about us are true.
- We can begin to overcome low self-esteem by challenging the accuracy of our negative core beliefs – our negative ideas about ourselves can *seem* true but they may not really *be* true.
- Another way of overcoming low self-esteem is to notice and build-up positive beliefs about ourselves.
- We can remind ourselves that negative thoughts and voice comments are not necessarily true.

- As we begin to overcome low self-esteem, we might notice that it is easier to dismiss the negative things the voices say and to pay the voices less attention.
- Overcoming low self-esteem is an important step on the road to overcoming distressing voices.

7

Changing our relationship with voices and other people

In Chapter 3 we spent some time thinking about the relationships that can exist between two people. We thought about how relationships involve give and take, and how giving and taking can be influenced by the power that one person has over the other and their proximity (closeness or distance) to each other. We identified that we often have two-way conversations with our voices, so we can think about relationships existing between ourselves and the voices we hear.

Relationships with distressing voices often leave us feeling dominated (as the voice uses its power to boss us around and try to control us) and intruded upon (as the voice does not respect our wishes for space and distance). We often respond by trying to distract ourselves from the voice and trying to create a bit of space for ourselves. If we can't escape the voice, we may respond by being aggressive and trying to fight back. Alternatively, we might give in and submit to the voice. In the long term, each of these ways of responding is unlikely to change the relationship with the voices we hear.

We also thought about the similarities between the relationships we have with voices and our relationships with family and friends. If we have positive relationships with our family and friends, this seems to have a positive effect upon our relationships with voices. On the other hand, negative relationships with family and friends can lead to relationships with voices being distressing. In some cases, very difficult relationships with family and friends can lead to people trying to escape from these relationships by investing in a relationship with voices, which may seem relatively safe and more predictable.

This chapter will take a step-by-step approach to changing our negative relationships with our voices, our friends and family, or both.

Step 1: Where to start – voices or other people? You choose!

If we want to change our relationships, where should we start? Should we begin by trying to change the relationship with our voices, or focus on relationships with family and friends? There is no right answer to this question. Positive change in one relationship is likely to have a positive influence on other relationships. Success leads to success as it generates confidence. When you successfully change a relationship, you will learn general principles that can be used again to change a different relationship. It is best to start where you are most likely to succeed.

This is likely to be a relationship that is difficult, but has the potential to change for the better if you make some changes in the way that you behave within the relationship. Before making the decision about which relationship to focus on, you will need to know your relationships really well. You might want to use Figure 20, overleaf, to make a list of the relationships that you find difficult, and put them into order according to the degree of difficulty and the likelihood of the relationship changing. You might want to discuss and create this list with someone who knows you well.

Figure 20: Mapping my relationships

Name of a person I have a difficult relationship with

____

____

____

How difficult is this relationship – on a scale of 0 'not difficult at all' to 10 'extremely difficult'

____

____

____

How likely is this relationship to change – on a scale of 0 'not at all likely' to 10 'extremely likely'

____

____

____

Name of a person I have a difficult relationship with

____

How difficult is this relationship – on a scale of 0 ‘not difficult at all’ to 10 ‘extremely difficult’

How likely is this relationship to change – on a scale of 0 ‘not at all likely’ to 10 ‘extremely likely’

Name of a person I have a difficult relationship with

How difficult is this relationship – on a scale of 0 ‘not difficult at all’ to 10 ‘extremely difficult’

How likely is this relationship to change – on a scale of 0 ‘not at all likely’ to 10 ‘extremely likely’

Name of a person I have a difficult relationship with

How difficult is this relationship – on a scale of 0 'not difficult at all' to 10 'extremely difficult'

How likely is this relationship to change – on a scale of 0 'not at all likely' to 10 'extremely likely'

Name of a person I have a difficult relationship with

How difficult is this relationship – on a scale of 0 'not difficult at all' to 10 'extremely difficult'

____

____

____

How likely is this relationship to change – on a scale of 0 'not at all likely' to 10 'extremely likely'

____

____

____

From the list you have made, choose the relationship that is most likely to change if you make an effort to change it. The relationship that Martin chose is described below.

Steps 2, 3 and 4 below will take you through the process of trying to change your relationships with the voice that you have chosen. If you have chosen to try to change a relationship with a family member or a friend, please go straight to Step 5.

Martin

Name of a person I have a difficult relationship with

Mother

How difficult is this relationship– on a scale of 0 to 10

7

How likely is this relationship to change – on a scale of 0 to 10

7

Name of a person I have a difficult relationship with

Voice of stepfather

How difficult is this relationship– on a scale of 0 to 10

10

How likely is this relationship to change – on a scale of 0 to 10

3

Name of a person I have a difficult relationship with

Sister

How difficult is this relationship– on a scale of 0 to 10

5

How likely is this relationship to change – on a scale of 0 to 10

7

Step 2: Changing relationships with voices

Making a decision to change your relationships with your voices is a very important first step. The next step is to investigate the relationship that you have chosen and get to know it as well as you can. This will involve thinking about the give and take within this relationship: how do you relate to your voice, and how does the voice relate to you? The obvious place to start is by focusing on the things that the voice says to you. Voices are often quite predictable and repetitive in what they say. Try using the following questions to remind you of what your voice says.

Exercise 1

Does your voice:

- Criticize you? If yes, write down what it says:

____

____

____

- Call you names? If yes, write down what it says:

____

____

____

- Tell you what to do? If yes, write down what it says:

____

____

____

- Comment on your activities? If yes, write down what it says:

____

____

____

- Talk about your past? If yes, write down what it says:

____

____

____

While answering these questions, you will have focused on the way that the voice relates to you. Focusing upon the voice may have seemed quite natural, but thinking about your role in the relationship may be harder. We often feel that we have no say in the relationships with our voices – it feels as if the relationships are all one-way traffic coming from the voices. But we are playing a role in the relationships – even if it doesn't feel as if this is so – and this is what we will be trying to change. Let's continue by using Figure 21 to think about the ways you respond to your voice. In the first column, write down one of the statements from your voice that you wrote down in Exercise 1 above.

Figure 21: How I respond to my voice

My voice says...

____

____

____

I feel ... angry, guilty, sad, upset, frightened

____

____

____

I say ... nothing, go away, swear, demand 'what do you want?'

____

____

____

I act by ... listening to music, going to sleep, getting drunk

____

____

____

My voice says...

____

____

____

I feel ... angry, guilty, sad, upset, frightened

____
____
____

I say ... nothing, go away, swear, demand 'what do you want?'

____
____
____

I act by ... listening to music, going to sleep, getting drunk

____
____
____

My voice says...

____
____
____

I feel ... angry, guilty, sad, upset, frightened

____
____
____

I say ... nothing, go away, swear, demand 'what do you want?'

I act by ... listening to music, going to sleep, getting drunk

How did you get on? Did you notice any patterns in how you respond to the voice? Did you notice if your responses were aggressive (fighting back) or passive (giving up)? Both these ways of responding are understandable, but they are unlikely to change your relationship with the voice in the long term. One way to change the relationship is to talk back in a more assertive way (this is not the same as being aggressive). By assertive, we mean talking and relating in ways that show respect for both yourself and the voice. Assertiveness involves communicating our feelings and opinions in an honest way that promotes a healthy view of ourselves and others. If you are trying to impose your feelings and opinions upon someone else, you are being aggressive rather than assertive. Aggression shows disrespect to the other person (or voice) by trying to dominate them and control their response. This might be how your voice relates to you. On the other hand, if you allow someone else to dominate your views, and if you give too much respect to what they feel and say, you are being passive rather than assertive. Passivity shows disrespect to yourself by allowing the other person (or voice) to dominate you. This might be how you relate to your voice. Being assertive is therefore a more balanced way of responding. To illustrate these differences, let's look at how Martin might respond to his voice. The three types of possible response are illustrated separately – passive, aggressive and assertive.

Martin responding passively

My voice says...

if you go out I will punish you

I feel...

frightened

I say...

okay, I will do as you say

I act by...

staying at home

Martin responding aggressively

My voice says...

if you go out I will punish you

I feel...

angry

I say...

you can't tell me what to do. Who the hell do you think you are?

I act by...

staying at home as the voice fights back and intimidates me

Martin responding assertively

My voice says...

if you go out I will punish you

I feel...

frightened

I say...

it's not okay for you to boss me around. I prefer to make my own decisions.

I act by...

I go out

Step 3: Becoming more assertive

Let's return to the relationship between you and your chosen voice and see what scope there is for you to be more assertive. We can do this by re-examining your responses to what your voice says, and trying to change this response into one that is more respectful to both yourself and the voice. Use the things that you previously wrote in Figure 21 to complete the first ***two*** columns of Table 3 overleaf.

How would you describe your typical response to your voices – aggressive or passive? A lot of people will respond in both ways – sometimes passively and sometimes aggressively. Now use the third column to label your response as either aggressive, assertive or passive.

If you rated your response as aggressive, you may have been using 'I' statements that left little room for the views of the voice, e.g. 'I must…'. You may also have been expressing your views as facts that cannot be disputed, e.g. 'What is going to happen is…'.

Table 3: Responding assertively to my voice

My voice says…

____

____

____

I respond by ... (feelings, actions, what I say)

____

____

____

Is my response passive, aggressive or assertive?

____

____

____

An assertive response would be...

____

____

____

My voice says...

____

____

____

I respond by ... (feelings, actions, what I say)

____

____

____

Is my response passive, aggressive or assertive?

____

____

____

An assertive response would be...

My voice says...

I respond by ... (feelings, actions, what I say)

Is my response passive, aggressive or assertive?

An assertive response would be...

If your response was a passive one, you may have been using 'I' statements that were hesitant and apologetic, e.g. 'I am ... er ... sorry to have to mention...'. You may also have been putting down and dismissing your views, e.g. 'I could be completely wrong but...'. A passive response may also involve not talking back to the voices at all.

When we are being assertive we will:

- Use 'I' statements such as:
  - * 'I prefer to...'
  - * 'I would like to...'
  - * 'I do not agree that...'
  - * 'I feel disappointed when...'
- Distinguish between fact and opinion:
  - * 'In my opinion...'
  - * 'As I understand it...'
  - * 'My experience is...'
- Constructively criticize without condemning:
  - * 'I feel disappointed when you...'
  - * 'I find it unacceptable when you...'
  - * 'I have noticed recently that...'

Let's return to the things that you previously wrote in Table 3. Use the fourth column to create and write an assertive response that uses clear 'I' statements. You might want to distinguish fact from opinion by questioning the accuracy of what the voice is saying. The voice may say something as if it is a fact (such as 'you are useless'), but this is only the opinion of the voice, which you have the right to question. Remember not to condemn the voice in the way that the voice is condemning you. Aggression is likely to provoke aggression, so express your feelings to the voice in a constructive and respectful way.

Having created an assertive response to one of your voice's common statements, the next step is to use the response when the voice is talking, and see what happens. This might feel like a big step, so it may be helpful to practise with someone you can trust, such as a friend, family member or mental health worker. This person can take on the role of the voice and say the statement commonly spoken by the voice, and you can respond with the assertive response that you have created. You will be interested in two things: 1) how did it feel when you gave the assertive response; 2) how did the other person feel when you spoke to them in this way, and how did they want to respond? Their feelings may act as a guide to how the voice will react to your assertive response. During this role-playing exercise, you will also need to be aware of your tone of voice, gestures and non-verbal communication. The following list describes some ways in which you can be assertive in a variety of verbal and non-verbal ways:

- Volume and tone of voice – a steady, warm tone will give an impression of confidence. You can stress key words to get across the strength of your feeling, without needing to shout.
- Pace of speech – clearly express your preference or opinion without hesitancy or stumbling. Fluent speech gives the impression of inner conviction and certainty in what you are saying.
- Maintaining eye contact – looking down or away is a sign of lack of confidence. Staring and glaring can be experienced as aggressive. Try to find a balance that communicates your confidence and invites a response.
- Facial expressions – your facial features should be consistent with what you are saying. For example, if you are pleased, you will smile; when frustrated you will frown. When being assertive your face will feel and look relaxed.
- Body movement and posture – an assertive posture is relaxed and confident, not slouched or bolt upright but somewhere in between. Don't fold your arms, point your finger or shake your fist, as these gestures can be experienced as defensive and aggressive.

Some of these non-verbal communications are more relevant to speaking with other people, rather than voices. But remember that we are trying to learn good habits for all types of relationships. Some of the above tips might also take a while to get the hang of. Be patient. Give yourself a break as you practise being assertive and gradually grow in confidence.

Having had a practice run or two, go back to your assertive response in Table 3 and make any changes to the response that might be needed. The next step will be to speak to the voice in this new, more assertive way.

Martin

My voice says...

if you go out I will punish you

I respond by ... (feelings, actions, speaking)

feeling frightened and staying at home

My response is passive or aggressive

passive

My assertive response is ...

it's not okay for you to boss me around. I prefer to make my own decisions. I would like to go out.

Step 4 – Having a different conversation

How did you get on? Did you talk to the voice in the new, assertive way? If yes, how did the voice respond? Voices often respond quite aggressively to assertiveness as they don't like you standing-up for yourself. The voice may also have tried to manipulate you by playing on your weaknesses and trying to undermine your confidence. And how did the conversation make you feel? Remember, relating is a two-way process, so the response of the voice to your assertiveness would have generated feelings and behaviours in you. Use Figure 22 below to describe and review the conversation that you had.

Figure 22: Reviewing my assertive response to my voice

My voice says...

____

____

____

My assertive response was...

____

____

____

My voice responded by...

This conversation made me feel...

My voice says...

My assertive response was...

My voice responded by...

This conversation made me feel...

My voice says...

My assertive response was...

My voice responded by...

This conversation made me feel...

Maybe you were not able to talk to the voice in an assertive way. Some of your beliefs about the voice (from Chapter 1) and yourself (from Chapter 2) may have taken away your confidence and provided you with excuses not to bother trying. For example ...

Beliefs about my voice:

- My voice is too powerful.
- My voice will harm me.
- My voice tells the truth.

Beliefs about myself:

- I am helpless.
- I am weak.
- I am too vulnerable.
- I am a failure.

You can use the techniques and guidance from Chapters 5 and 6 to help you to question the accuracy of these beliefs about your voice and yourself. For example, try exploring the evidence that means that the beliefs are not completely true all of the time.

Once you have tried responding to one of the voice's comments in an assertive way, two things are really important. First, practise. Doing something for the first time is often difficult and a bit scary, but it gets a little easier each time you try. So be sure to use your assertive response each time the voice makes these particular comments. Second, spread your assertiveness to other conversations you have with the voice. Use the figures and tables above to identify other comments that the voice regularly says and how you usually respond, and create a more assertive response instead. Practise using this assertive response until it feels like second nature. And keep track of how you feel, both in the moment of responding assertively, and more generally. The next step is to speak to other voices and people in this more assertive manner.

Martin

My voice says...

if you go out I will punish you

My assertive response was...

it's not okay for you to boss me around. I prefer to make my own decisions. I would like to go out.

My voice responded by...

shouting loudly at me

The conversation made me feel...

anxious, but also determined to stand up to this bullying voice

My voice says...

you're weak and pathetic and can't stand up for yourself

My assertive response was...

I don't agree that I'm weak. What evidence do you have to support your view?

My voice responded by...

repeating itself by saying that I was weak and pathetic

The conversation made me feel...

brave: I stood up to the voice and it didn't know what to say

Step 5: Relationships with other people

In Chapter 3 we learnt that distressing relationships with voices often go hand in hand with distressing relationships with family and friends. Return to Figure 20 in Step 1 and find the names of people that you struggle to get along with. Being assertive with these people and developing balanced relationships with them is really important, and is likely to affect both your relationships with your voices and your views of yourself.

Take the name of someone from Figure 20 and use Figure 23 (taken from Step 2) to identify a negative comment that they often make – and your usual response.

Figure 23: How I respond to other people

The other person says...

____

____

____

I feel ... angry, guilty, sad, upset, frightened

I say ... nothing, go away, swear, ask 'what do you want?'

I act by ... listening to music, going to sleep, getting drunk

The other person says...

I feel ... angry, guilty, sad, upset, frightened

I say ... nothing, go away, swear, ask 'what do you want?'

I act by ... listening to music, going to sleep, getting drunk

The other person says...

I feel ... angry, guilty, sad, upset, frightened

I say ... nothing, go away, swear, ask 'what do you want?'

I act by ... listening to music, going to sleep, getting drunk

Then follow Step 3 to create a new, more assertive response. To begin with, you might want to practise using this new, assertive response with someone you trust. When you feel ready, use the guidance from Step 4 to help you to try out the assertive response and see what happens. Make sure you pay attention to your tone of voice and non-verbal communication. These things may have seemed less important when you were responding to the voice but, when relating to people who are physically in your presence, they become vital aspects of communication that back up the words you are saying. There is little point in using assertive words if every other aspect of your communication comes across as either aggressive or passive.

Martin

My mum says...

you need to pull yourself together

My assertive response was...

I don't agree. I am doing okay at the moment.

My mum responded by...

saying nothing, she seemed to be lost for words

The conversation made me feel...

chuffed with myself for being assertive

What's changing?

In Chapter 3, we said it was important to change your relationships if you can, rather than rely on coping strategies that may not benefit you in the longer term. If you have tried some of the techniques from this chapter to help you change your relationships, and feel that you were successful, in what ways are you now benefitting?

You might want to revisit the Self-Esteem Scale that you completed in Chapter 2. Answer the questions again. Have any of your responses changed for the better? Do you feel that you have more worth and respect for yourself? You can also revisit the questionnaires that you completed in Chapter 3 about the power and intrusiveness of your voices. Do you notice if any of your responses have changed, hopefully for the better? For example, are your voices being less dominant and intrusive?

Martin changing his relationships

We saw in Chapter 3 that Martin had a difficult relationship with the voice of his stepfather who bullied him and made him feel weak and vulnerable. This led to Martin responding passively to the voice, and strengthened his negative feelings about himself. After using the techniques set out in this chapter, Martin was able to be assertive with the voice of his stepfather. He stood up to the voice, questioned the accuracy of the voice's put-downs and felt more positive about himself as a result. Martin also tried to be more assertive with members of his family and was proud of himself for trying to change his relationships for the better, which in turn boosted his self-esteem.

Summary

In this chapter, we have seen how we can play an active role in our relationships with our voices, and with friends and family. We can change our way of relating in an aggressive or passive way to being assertive, which will help us to have relationships that are equal and two-way. Assertive responses involve being respectful of both ourselves and the voice/other person. If we are able to respond assertively within our relationships with other people and our voices, we are likely to notice an improvement in our self-esteem, and changes in the way that the voice/person relates to us.

Key points

- We can try to change our relationships with our voices and our relationships with family and friends. It doesn't matter where we start – positive change in one relationship is likely to have a positive influence on other relationships.

- Once you have decided which relationship you want to change, it is important to investigate the relationship and get to know it as well as you can.
- It is important to notice patterns in the way that you respond within this relationship – are you being aggressive or passive?
- You need to change your responses into ones that are assertive – which respect both yourself and the voice/person you are relating to.
- Your assertive responses will need to use clear 'I' statements, and distinguish fact from opinion (for instance, by questioning the accuracy of what is being said to you).
- When you are responding assertively you will also need to be aware of your tone of voice, gestures and nonverbal communication.
- Voices/other people may not appreciate your attempts at being assertive and may respond negatively.
- Practise is important, so be sure to use your assertive responses every time you have conversations with this voice/person.
- As your responses become more assertive you may feel that you have more worth and respect for

yourself. You may also notice that the voice/person is being less dominant and intrusive.

Part Four

Looking to the Future

8

Moving forwards

The diagram below shows the different ways in which we have learnt to understand and overcome distressing voices during the course of this book.

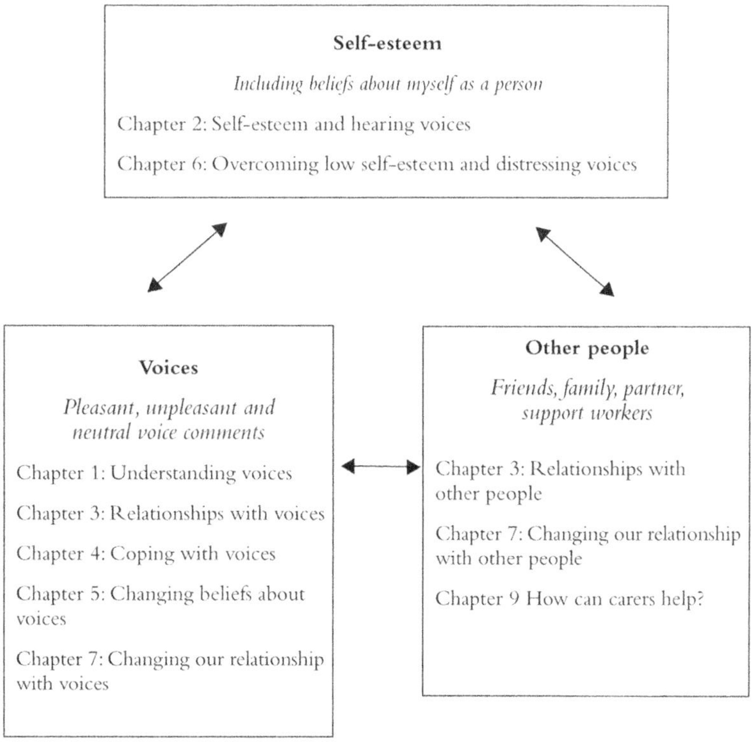

In this book, we have seen that hearing voices is not an unusual experience – lots of people hear voices. In Chapter 1, we saw that some people who hear voices are not particularly distressed by their experience and can find hearing voices pleasant and comforting. However, other people can feel very distressed at hearing voices; common reactions can include feeling depressed, anxious and angry. So, hearing voices is, in itself, not a problem – the problem arises when voices cause a lot of distress and when voices interfere with how we want to live our lives.

Because hearing voices is itself not a problem, the focus of this book has been on how to overcome *distress* at hearing voices, rather than to focus on how to get rid of the voices. Not everyone wants to get rid of voices (some people actually like hearing voices). Even if we would like to get rid of them, it is not always possible to stop voices completely. What *is* possible is to reduce feelings of distress in response to voices, and to stop letting the voices get in the way of what we want to do in our lives. The ideas in this book, therefore, are aimed at overcoming distress at hearing voices and at finding ways of leading our lives the way we want to lead them – and without the voices getting too much in the way of what we want to do.

There are different ways of overcoming distressing voices and this book has introduced a range of techniques and ideas to begin to do that. Hopefully you will have found all the ideas in this book helpful, or you may have found some of the ideas more helpful than others. There is no right way to overcome distressing voices, you can choose the ideas that you find most helpful and focus on these. The aim of this book has been to offer some easy-to-use resources for people who may have found voice-hearing too hard to deal with. We will now summarize the different ways that we have looked at for overcoming distressing voices.

Coping with voices

In Chapter 4 we looked at a number of practical ways of coping with distressing voices. The ideas in Chapter 4 can be a good place to start, as it can help to reduce our feelings of distress and help prepare us for challenging our beliefs about voices.

Identifying and changing our beliefs about voices

In Chapter 1 we saw that whether or not we feel distressed by voices depends in large part on what we believe and think about them. If we believe that the voices don't have much control or power, and if we don't believe the unpleasant things the voices say, then we might not feel particularly bothered. If, on the other hand, we believe that voices have power and control over us, and if we tend to believe that the unpleasant voice comments are true, then we are much more likely to feel distressed. We saw from Martin and Sarah's stories in Chapter 1 that what we think and believe about voices can make a big difference to how we feel and how we live our lives.

So, what we believe about voices is important. In Chapter 5 we looked at a step-by-step approach to identifying and challenging unhelpful beliefs about voices. This chapter looked at ways of noticing evidence that voices do not always have control and power over us, and that voices do not always speak the truth. If we begin to change our beliefs about voices, and begin to believe that voices do not have much power or control and that voices do not always speak the truth, then we might find that we begin to feel less distressed by the things the voices say.

Overcoming low self-esteem

In Chapter 2 we saw that hearing distressing voices often goes hand in hand with having a low opinion of ourselves and having negative beliefs about ourselves ('core beliefs'). This happens because difficult life experiences, particularly in childhood, make it more likely that we will develop low self-esteem, and also make it more likely that we will hear voices. Having low self-esteem also makes it more likely that we will believe any unpleasant things the voices say about us. The important point in this chapter was to find out that although our negative core beliefs can *feel* true, they rarely *are* true.

In Chapter 6 we learnt ways of identifying and challenging negative self-esteem beliefs. The ideas in this chapter helped us to notice negative core beliefs we have about ourselves and led us through ways of gathering evidence to help us re-assess the accuracy of these beliefs. At the same time, we looked at the fact that negative core beliefs can be hard to shift, particularly if they have been around since we were young children. Because of this, we then looked at noticing and building up positive, alternative core beliefs about ourselves. Using the same step-by-step approach, we found out how to carefully and slowly gather evidence that would help to support a more positive view of ourselves.

Relationships with voices

Chapter 3 introduced us to the idea that we can think about having a relationship with voices in much the same way as we have relationships with the people in our lives. Our relationships with people involve give and take and can be considered in terms of power (who, if anyone, holds most power in the relationship and how do they use this power?) and closeness (how close or distant are we in the relationship and who decides how close we are?). We can also think about voices in this way. Where does the power lie in our relationship with the voices? If the voices have more power, do they use this power to dominate and bully us? How close or distant is our relationship with the voices? Are the voices too close and intrusive? Voices that dominate, bully and intrude can lead us to respond aggressively and passively towards them. Chapter 7 led us through ways of changing our relationship with the voices so that the relationship can become more balanced. By being assertive with the voices, we can begin to feel as if we have some power and control within the relationship, and create some space to help us do the things that we want to do.

Relationships with other people

In Chapter 3 we also talked about relationships with people in terms of power and closeness. We saw that the kinds of relationships we develop with voices might be quite similar to the kinds of relationships we develop with important people in our lives. So, if we tend to be passive in our relationships with the people in our lives, then we might find that we respond passively to voices. Because of this, in Chapter 7, we looked at ways of changing our relationships with other people, particularly by becoming more assertive. As a result, we might feel more confident and assertive towards the voices.

Finally, in Chapter 9 we will look at ways that important people such as friends, family and support workers can help us to overcome distressing voices. We all depend on other people for our well-being, and Chapter 9 looks at practical ways in which other people can help us in overcoming distressing voices. Important, trusted people in our lives might also help us to work through the other chapters in this book.

Moving beyond voices – Martin's story

We first met Martin in Chapter 1, where we were shown that he was distressed by hearing voices and that voices stopped him from doing the things he wanted to do in his life. Martin believed that his voices had power and control over him, which meant that when the voices made threatening comments Martin would stay at home rather than risk going out. His beliefs that the voices had power and control over him were linked to his feelings of low self-esteem and his negative core belief that he was weak and vulnerable. Because he saw himself as weak and vulnerable he tended to believe that other people – and the voices – were more in control and more powerful than he was. From this, we saw that Martin had a relationship with the voices that was passive; the voices had the upper hand. The more passively Martin related to the voices, the more powerful they seemed to be. We can see from Martin's story how his beliefs about the voices, his negative core beliefs about himself, and the relationship he had with the voices and with other people, were all connected and led to a vicious cycle:

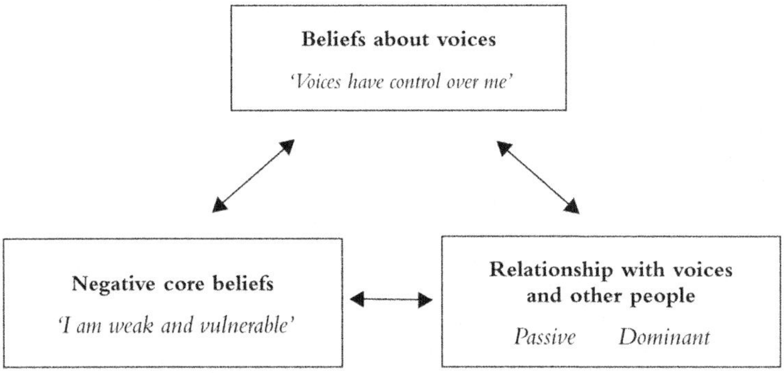

This is how things were for Martin before trying the techniques in this book. How are things for Martin now? By using the ideas presented in Chapter 4, Martin learnt to cope with distressing voices in practical ways that helped to reduce his feelings of anxiety. He listened to music to distract himself from his voices, talked on Facebook to stay in touch with friends, cooked and cleaned around the home, and spoke to a mental health worker about his voices. By learning how to manage his feelings of anxiety, Martin felt able to tackle his beliefs about the voices (see Chapter 5). He was able to identify that one of his core beliefs was that 'the voices have control over me', and then carefully and slowly gather evidence and experiences to show that this belief did not stand up in the face of the evidence. By carefully looking at the evidence, Martin came to realize that the voices didn't always have control over him and, because of this, he began to feel a little better and began to consider doing more things in his life. He then began to work on his negative core belief 'I am weak and vulnerable' (see Chapter 6). He was able to notice and write down evidence that challenged the accuracy of this belief, thus he began to believe it less strongly. Martin was also able to notice a positive belief about himself – that he was likeable – and he began to notice and write down evidence that this was true. Once he'd been doing this for a few weeks, he had gained the confidence to start doing things differently and decided to contact old friends he had lost touch with.

Martin took these ideas further by exploring the way in which he related to the voices (see Chapter 7). He realized that he'd related to them in a passive way, just like he related to the important people in his life. Martin practised acting assertively with the voice of his stepfather, and because this worked out well, he was able to begin to practise acting more assertively with his mother.

Martin's story is similar to one we have heard many times and, like Martin, many of the people we have worked with using the ideas in this book have been able to begin to overcome distressing voices. Here are some things that the people we've worked with have said after following the ideas we've introduced to them.

People told us that they had changed their beliefs about voices, one person said:

> *It's made me stronger, not to believe everything the voices say.*

Another person told us about their changed relationship with voices:

> *One thing I learnt was that I could take a stand against the voices and not necessarily allow them to overtake me – to control me.*

When it comes to building up positive self-esteem someone we worked with said:

> *Voices still tell me about my bad points, but I've realized I've still got good points as well. The important thing I've realized is that I have good points.*

When it comes to relationships with other people, one of the people we worked with said:

> *I think I'm more open now. I tend to talk to people a lot more. Whereas before I was quite reclusive, now I go to my parents' quite often, which is something I didn't do before. I tend to phone my mum quite a lot now and I go out with friends a lot more, which is again something I didn't do before.*

These comments show how it is possible to begin to overcome distressing voices – we can change our beliefs about voices, change how we relate to voices, build up our self-esteem and work to change our relationships with important people in our lives.

Moving forwards

One of the people we worked with said:

> *I feel that I am a person at the end of it, even despite these voices.*

To us, this comment captures what this book is all about. Hearing voices, as we saw in Chapter 1, can lead to a great deal of distress and disturbance to our quality of life. This can mean that we become lost in listening to voices or arguing with voices, or it can mean that we become preoccupied with trying to avoid and ignore voices. If we end up spending most of our time thinking about (or trying hard *not* to think about) voices, we can all too easily lose sight of who we are. The same person who said that they now feel like a person, despite the voices, said that in the past:

> *I had been beginning to lose my identity, just seeing myself constantly as an ill person.*

Working through the ideas in this book is about overcoming distressing voices to make way for a new identity – a sense of self that is no longer defined in terms of hearing voices.

Where next?

Once we have begun to overcome distressing voices, this can create room in our lives for doing things that bring us pleasure and a sense of achievement. Using the space below, you might want to write down what you would be doing if it wasn't for distressing voices. This might include things that would bring you pleasure (hobbies, activities, socializing), things that would give you a sense of achievement (doing a course, something creative) and things that would give you a sense of meaning and purpose (helping other people, voluntary work).

If distressing voices were not around I would be doing:

1. ______
2. ______
3. ______
4. ______
5. ______

Looking at your list, would it be possible to start doing any of these things now, even if voices are still around? Might it be possible, using the ideas you've found helpful in this book, to make a start on some of the things in the list? It is important not to put pressure on yourself to do more than you feel able to do right now – so, if it feels possible to do something on the list, you might want to choose the thing that feels most manageable to do right now. You may also want to take just a first step towards doing something on the list. So if you've written 'get a paid job' but this feels too difficult at the moment, then a first step might be looking for voluntary work, perhaps in a local charity shop for a few hours per week.

What is possible? By starting to do the things we enjoy or that give us a sense of personal achievement, even if voices are still around, we might find more evidence that the voices don't always have control and that they don't always speak the truth. We might find more evidence to challenge the negative core beliefs we hold about ourselves and to strengthen positive self-esteem beliefs – and we might have plenty of opportunities to practice acting assertively in our relationships with other people.

Some of the people we have worked with who have heard distressing voices have since started socializing more with friends and family, made new friends, started new relationships, begun adult-education classes, gone to college or university, begun doing voluntary work or found a paying job, joined a gym or a walking group, and many other things. As we saw from Sarah's story and from the survey by Marius Romme and Sandra Escher, hearing voices does not have to be a barrier to doing the things we want to do in our lives.

Part Five

Carers and Distressing Voices

9

How can carers help?

When someone you know and care about hears distressing voices, it can be very confusing for family and friends. Initially, it is usually the case that you don't actually know that the person is hearing voices – and this may also be very confusing. People who hear voices often initially assume that other people can hear what is being said – but are then surprised, puzzled or even annoyed when other people don't respond to what they're hearing. As realization begins to dawn on them that it's possible that you can't hear the voices, the person may check with you if you can hear what is being said. If this realization doesn't happen, however, it can affect your relationship as the person you care for may become more distant and even angry with you.

People who hear voices usually begin to come to some understanding that the voices they hear are not heard by others, but this doesn't always happen or can take quite a while to emerge. The following example of Gary and his carers illustrates these issues.

Gary's story

John and Sue have cared for their son, Gary, for six years since he was first diagnosed with schizophrenia. He had been using marijuana and amphetamines for two or three years prior to the diagnosis. This had led to friction within the family, but the emergence of severe mental health problems was still a shock. Gary's family had been trying to get him help with his drug-taking – because he was becoming more and more isolated – but he didn't believe he needed help and there seemed to be no one able to advise them what to do.

The first time Gary was admitted to hospital he was very confused and agitated. He was demanding to be let free, talking rapidly and incoherently, and was praying for mercy. He gradually improved during his time on the ward and eventually returned home, but he seemed to remain preoccupied, often talking to himself. He would go out to see some of his old friends, but would usually return home under the influence of drugs or alcohol. This caused arguments and he would be even more irritable the next day.

Over the years, with discussion with mental health staff and a local family's group, John and Sue managed to negotiate with Gary the boundaries of what was and what was not acceptable behaviour. These boundaries were not always adhered to but he at least seemed to make some attempts to comply.

It turned out that Gary was hearing voices, which could be very distressing to him, accusing him of doing bad things and telling him to harm himself. He believed they were the voices of the devil and would talk to them for much of the day.

Gary's drug-use gradually reduced as his friends moved on. He also began to gain some understanding of how his voices were directly related to the problems he was experiencing and, therefore, it began to make sense to him as to how psychiatric medication might help. He also began to make the link with his early drug-use.

John and Sue had learnt more about the nature of voice-hearing from their own reading, and in joint therapy sessions with Gary and a therapist who worked with them for a few months. If Gary got agitated, they could ask him directly if the voices were troubling him, and work out with him if any of his usual tactics for dealing with them might be helpful.

Gary continued to talk to the voices, which could be distracting and annoying for his family, so they agreed that if it was a problem to them they would ask him if he minded going into another room – and maybe listen to music or play a computer game until the voices settled down. Both Gary and his family recognized that distress and agitation, especially arguments, just made the situation worse. By Gary's family identifying when he was talking to the voices, this helped Gary in turn to learn when he was talking to them. Just as sometimes people talk to themselves when on their own and preoccupied, so Gary didn't always realize he was talking back to his voices. Also, what he said could be rude or very strange and this led on occasions to arguments in the street and in pubs. Gentle prompting from John and Sue helped Gary, until the voices became less and less of a problem for him.

> Gary still hears voices but they are not as distressing and he is controlling his responses to them well. It has meant that he has become able to cope better for himself – he has moved into his own flat. He is making some friends who don't use drugs and is thinking about what other activities he might develop. John and Sue keep in regular contact but are beginning to get a life of their own.

Seeking help

It may become clear that the person you care for needs help because of the effect the voices have on them, or because of behaviour changes such as stopping activities, becoming isolated, or saying things that don't appear to make sense. However, when someone starts to hear voices, it can be very difficult to identify that there is something wrong. At what point in someone's worsening difficulties or increasing distress, is help needed? The problems that the person is experiencing are confusing and not well understood by most people but can be clarified and, to a large extent, overcome with the appropriate help. Such help may come through contact with a family doctor or directly through a mental health service.

If it is a friend or relative of yours who is experiencing difficulties, you will want them to come to understand that they need to meet someone to discuss the voice-hearing experiences and learn ways of understanding and coping with what is happening. The person you care for may be very fearful of what the voices are saying or threatening – often they may find that the voices tell them not to seek help, not to believe or trust anyone, etc. It can be very confusing for the person hearing voices if it seems to them that someone is speaking but then that person can't be found when looked for. The person hearing the voices may become paranoid and try to explain what is happening as 'someone out to get them' – maybe blaming neighbours or even the government. The person may start to fear that they are going mad and actively resist this, or anything implying that this might be the case – for example, being advised to see a doctor, psychiatrist or mental health worker, and especially taking medication.

Reasons for voices

In most cases, the person hearing the voices – perhaps a friend or relative you care about – will have been feeling stressed before the voices start, and this will have contributed to the voice-hearing. The stress caused by the experience of hearing voices can then very often make things worse. It can be helpful to acknowledge that the person has been having a hard time and this can be used as a reason to seek help. 'Everybody gets stressed ... it's just the way we react that can differ' – voices and confusion being alongside getting anxious, depressed, drinking too much, overworking, etc. So, you could say to the person that, 'we need to do something to help reduce the stress you are experiencing and help you cope with it as effectively as possible'. It is important not to convey to the person that you think – or even that they think you think (!) – that they are inadequate in any way, but rather that we can all experience problems from time to time and that there is help available. Voice-hearing doesn't mean your friend or relative is mad.

As we saw in Chapter 1 of this book, many people – including many well-known people – have heard voices, especially when under stress. Stress in one form or another is usually a factor in people starting to hear distressing voices. The stress may be obvious and due to bullying or work pressures, etc. There may then be a straightforward way of managing it that may stop the voices, or at least reduce them, e.g. stop the bullying or take some time off work and review how to manage the stress involved. It may still be worth getting some help to keep things settled.

However, it may not be immediately obvious what caused the voices to start, particularly when the voices seem to have gradually emerged as a problem. Voice-hearing can be triggered by any number of circumstances such as the pressures of trying to find or maintain a job, develop friendships or relationships, or moving to a new environment such as going to college or university. These may not seem like particularly stressful events, after all, most people experience these things without developing problems, but sometimes a combination of factors, even some of which arise from childhood, can make the stress become overwhelming – and thus beliefs and voices can develop that are disturbing and interfere with life.

Strengths and vulnerabilities

Some vulnerability to voices may come from the way the brain works, but there is no evidence yet that there is a specific malfunction that can be seen under a microscope or using other brain-scanning techniques, nor does there seem to be a specific chemical abnormality that causes voice-hearing. The issue of genetic transmission is also not straightforward. There is evidence that people who hear voices are more likely than others to have members of their family who also experience voices and other associated experiences, but this is the same for most mental health problems and many physical ones also. The determining factor may be ways of coping and interacting with other people – personality – which does seem to be genetically transmitted although with a lot of influence from people's life circumstances. We are like our parents in many ways – whether we like it or not.

In Chapter 2 we discovered how difficult life circumstances can have a big impact upon self-esteem, and how low self-esteem often goes hand in hand with people who hear distressing voices. In Chapter 6 we saw how self-esteem can be worked upon to help people who hear distressing voices to see themselves more positively.

Trauma

The issues of trauma and psychosis are complex and this is particularly the case for carers. It is very important to make clear that many people who hear distressing voices have grown up in loving and supportive families. Of course, some will have had experiences that have been damaging – the person you care about may or may not have had such experiences. If they *have* had early childhood traumatic experiences – bullying or physical, sexual or emotional abuse, they may have had these experiences before they came into your care, e.g. if you fostered or adopted them – or the experiences may have happened when they were temporarily under someone else's care. It occasionally happens that someone conceals such experiences but it is unlikely that they would hide their experience from a carer indefinitely – although it may come out a number of years later and sometimes to someone else.

If the person who is hearing the voices has experienced traumatic events early in life, it can clearly be difficult for carers to know the best way to provide support. They may even feel that they have provided tremendous support to the individual yet feel accused of not doing enough or even causing the problems. If that is the case, you as a carer are probably going to need support from others yourself.

It may be that the person can't or won't discuss the exact details but instead vaguely refers to the fact that 'something happened' at some stage. They may find it difficult to talk about some events to a family member but may be able to talk to a therapist at a later stage.

It is distressing if someone you care about has bad experiences that are out of your control or perhaps occurred when you were not around, e.g. this can happen when families separate or if you've adopted or fostered the person you care for, or they've come to live with you with a new partner. Such issues, though, can be very important and have a major effect on someone's life and the way, for example, that they experience hearing voices.

Sometimes when someone is very distressed, the confusion can lead to accusations against family members that are not based on real events. This can be incredibly stressful and distressing for all concerned and carers may need a lot of support, advice and understanding to cope. Organizations such as Rethink Mental Illness and MIND in the UK, and similar organizations elsewhere, may provide this advice and help. Mental health services also need to be available for carers, and often have workers specifically allotted to work with and support them.

Voices often relate directly to stressful events. They may actually sound just like the person who was responsible for what happened, e.g. a school bully, and be saying the sort of threatening and abusive things that were said during the actual events. In this case, it can seem to the person who is experiencing these voices that the aggressor is really there – or close by, or by some magical or supernatural process is communicating with them. The power that the abusive person had over them may seem very real and the voice-hearer may feel compelled to do what the voices command, and can be very frightened to go against anything that the voice says.

Drugs

Sometimes a person hears voices because they have taken certain recreational drugs – especially amphetamines, cocaine or marijuana. Usually, for this to happen, the drug-use has been prolonged. The initial experiences of hearing voices and feeling suspicious (paranoia) stop as the direct effects of the drugs wear off, but sometimes the voices continue even when the drugs are not being taken. So, where drugs are involved it can become quite complicated. Occasionally the experience can be so distressing that the person spontaneously stops using drugs or just comes to a realization that drugs are harmful – but, as mentioned, even after stopping the drugs sometimes the voices continue and assistance is needed in terms of psychological and drug treatment.

Unfortunately, more often than not the drug-use continues. There are positive experiences that the person gets from drugs, especially relaxation, which can ironically reduce the severity of the voices. So the cause of the voices can sometimes actually have a relaxing effect. Also, the person may find peer pressure from other friends taking drugs – and pressure from suppliers – difficult to resist. Finding ways of managing voices more effectively is the goal – drugs overall will keep the problem going but some sort of help to reduce the voices' intensity and stress needs to go in their place – which is where a family doctor or mental health services can help. The objective will be to find alternative ways of relaxing and to develop a circle of friends who can help with staying away from drugs.

Drug-use is a problem in making voices worse but it can also trigger other behaviour, e.g. stealing, bullying and aggression, which can be major problems in their own right. Distinguishing between behaviour related to hearing voices and what is 'bad' behaviour can be difficult. 'Bad' behaviour can mean being selfish, rude or demanding – not directly due to 'illness'. It is certainly important not to approve of behaviour that is negatively affecting others, even where voices are involved. It may be necessary to encourage the person hearing the voices to resist what the voices say to them. On the rare occasions where the law is broken, the involvement of the police may be necessary. It can be very difficult to balance the views and opinions of the voice-hearer, carers, psychiatrists and mental health staff, and, occasionally, the police. This kind of extreme situation can only be helped by constructive discussion.

Responding when someone is hearing voices

How should you respond when you know someone is hearing voices? There are some basic things that are important in developing a good relationship with anyone. These are:

- Empathizing – trying to be understanding. It probably doesn't help to say 'I know how you feel' unless you've had very similar experiences yourself. Something along the lines of 'that sounds upsetting or unpleasant' may be better.
- Acceptance – it can be frightening and confusing when someone you know starts to hear voices but it is important to remember that the person you care for is not now a different person but the same

person with a new problem. Accepting people as who they are, and offering support, can make recovery more likely. It is also important not to look down on the person you care for, or give up hope for the future, as there is more and more happening in terms of new research and developing treatments to make life more acceptable and recovery more possible for people who hear distressing voices. Timing and short- and long-term expectations are important – being too demanding or having unrealistic expectations of the voice-hearer can put them under pressure and set progress back. On the other hand, going at an appropriate pace and being encouraging can be very effective.

- Being non-judgemental – try not to use words that criticize or judge, e.g. avoid statements such as 'this is your punishment for taking drugs' or 'you should do this ... or you must try that...' expressions. It is quite reasonable to ask – 'Do you think the drugs or some other experience might have started this? What do you think might help?' But it is also important not to repeatedly harp on about 'what the person has done wrong' – once you've got your message across.

- Balancing warmth and space – being warm towards someone can really help. Even when you may have had arguments and upsets – encouraging, smiling or looking sad where appropriate can really help. That doesn't mean forcing expressions but trying to naturally respond to the person in the situation, accepting that they are struggling – although, as mentioned before, being able to set and describe limits on their behaviour if it is disturbing. However, you may need to consider maintaining the personal space that the person wants – they may want you to give them time on their own – and also not ask too often how they are feeling. Getting the balance right means talking with them about how best you can help. Not doing too much for the person you care for – encouraging activity and independence – can be best. Sometimes you may be put under emotional pressure to provide money for drugs or alcohol – it is very unlikely that this will help the situation in the long or even short term.

Hearing a distressing voice can be like being in a difficult relationship (see Chapter 3). You can help by offering a supportive relationship that provides an example of how a relationship can be positive (see Chapter 7).

If the experience of distressing voices is quite new to you or the person experiencing them, asking simple questions about the experiences might help you understand these better – and it might clarify things for the voice-hearer too.

- What is upsetting you?

The person may be able to tell you, but he/she might be frightened or ashamed of the voices and what the voices are saying – thus you may not get a response.

If you think the person you care for might be hearing voices, or you are told directly that this is so, it might be worth persisting by gently prompting responses.

- Are you hearing someone talk or shout? Is it like speech? Like someone talking to you?

The voice-hearer may be able to explain that it is like someone speaking to them or maybe it is different in some ways.

- Where does it seem to be coming from?

It might be helpful to work out what is causing the sounds – sometimes it is a misinterpretation of sounds from a machine, e.g. from a refrigerator, or sounds through a wall or window. Compare experiences – e.g. saying that you can hear a hum but not spoken words or you can't hear anything but you do accept that he/she is hearing something.

- What are you hearing?

The voice-hearer may not be able to tell you if it is particularly unpleasant or may just tell you generally what is being said, e.g. 'they keep on insulting me or are swearing at me'. It is not necessary to know all the details – the person may be trying to protect you from disturbing or abusive comments.

If what's said is unpleasant, it is good to just recognize that, e.g. 'that sounds nasty' or 'distressing' or maybe 'strange' and to be supportive.

You may then ask:

- Do you recognize who it is?

Sometimes people hearing voices do not recognize the voice or voices, while sometimes the voice does refer to someone known, or sometimes to someone off the TV or from a film. The person hearing the voices may also have developed a name for the voice, or a label – such as the Devil or God – and may want to say more about the experiences and how they relate to other experiences and beliefs. Sometimes voices are believed to have spiritual origins, or predict the future, or be part of a conspiracy. Making room for the person to discuss these beliefs can be very helpful as it enables the experience to be shared. At least initially, it is usually best not to try to contradict what is said or express disbelief, or even point out contradictions in what is said. Giving the person space to express their views can often help towards a better understanding of them and what is happening. Sometimes the person will see that there are inconsistencies in what the voices say and with other experiences. If they ask if you believe the voices too, initially it is worth giving the benefit of the doubt, as sometimes the beliefs expressed or the things the voices say reflect some real experiences or events in some way.

As time progresses, it will become clearer that the experiences are hallucinatory – not real – and it may become appropriate to gently express this view if asked, whilst at the same time not being dismissive of the person hearing the voices.

What can voices say?

Voices may tell the person hearing them what to do and this can be disturbing for the person and for their family, especially if the voices are telling them to harm themselves or other people. It is certainly important that you encourage the person to discuss this with the family doctor (if they are not yet in touch with a mental health service). It is very unusual for people to obey the commands of the voices in a way that endangers themselves or others – in some ways, the voices are often expressing the thoughts and fears of the person hearing them and, because of this, it is possible to take measures to improve the situation and safeguard against these fears. But it is still important to see that any risks are managed properly early on, with expert advice and care.

Sometimes voices are abusive and this can be hard to take, especially when it goes on for long periods, day after day. Often it reflects how the voice-hearer feels about themselves – and if the person didn't feel that way when the voices started, the repetition can almost 'brainwash' them into believing what is said. Difficulties can start when people are depressed and maybe thinking negative things about themselves, with the thoughts turning gradually into voices over time.

Dealing with these sorts of voices can be difficult, but family and friends can really help by supporting, encouraging and being positive about their friend or relative – criticism is certainly not helpful. Helping the person you care for to see the positive things about themselves – offering reminders of achievements in the present and in the past, despite the voices – can be useful. Engaging them in an activity and helping them to focus on other things can also be helpful. We describe in Chapter 4 the sort of coping strategies that can help and assist.

Carers need support too!

Hearing voices is an experience that can be difficult to understand and respond to in a helpful way, especially when you've had no contact with anybody with such problems before. People's experience of voices can be mixed – there are a lot of people who hear voices but don't seek help because they find it to be a positive experience. There are others who learn to cope effectively with the voices; for others, the voices come and go – and perhaps go altogether. The person hearing voices can benefit significantly from the support that you can offer them, but you need to make sure that you use any available supports yourself as well. To find out more about what support may be available in your area, try asking your local mental health services. They will usually provide a carer's support worker or links to agencies that can help (e.g. Rethink Mental Illness and MIND – see website addresses at the end of this book).

Summary and key points

The experience of hearing voices can be very confusing and upsetting for the person who hears them. It can also be difficult for the people who care for the voice-hearer. Things that seem to help are:

- Trying to generate an understanding of how voices develop – and particularly how they've developed for the person you are caring for.
- Working out how to respond most helpfully when the voices are causing distress or other disturbance, e.g. when the voice-hearer is answering back to the voices.
- Helping the voice-hearer find ways of coping with their voices.
- Finding sources of advice and support for yourself and any other family members who might benefit.

Useful organizations

British Association for Behavioural & Cognitive Psychotherapies (BABCP)

BABCP is the lead organization for CBT in the UK. Here you can find details of all officially accredited cognitive-behavioural therapists.

Website: www.babcp.com

International Society for Psychological and Social Approaches to Psychosis (ISPS)

ISPS promotes psychological treatments for people who experience psychosis (e.g. hallucinations and delusions), and greater understanding of the psychological and social causes of psychosis.

Website: www.isps.org

National Institute for Health and Clinical Excellence (NICE)

NICE uses the best available research evidence to make recommendations to the NHS about which treatments to provide. Recommendations about CBT for schizophrenia were published in 2002 and 2009.

Website: www.nice.org.uk

Hearing Voices Network (HVN) (UK)

HVN offers information, support and understanding to people who hear voices and those who support them, e.g. promoting, developing and supporting self-help groups, and a telephone line that gives information and help.

Website: www.hearing-voices.org

Email: nhvn@hotmail.co.uk

Intervoice – online international community for hearing voices

Intervoice is The International Community for Hearing Voices. It undertakes training, education and research. Online resources include a discussion forum and links to hearing voices groups worldwide.

Website: www.intervoiceonline.org

MIND, for better mental health

Mind helps people to take control over their mental health by providing information and advice, training programmes, grants and services through a network of local Mind associations.

Website: www.mind.org.uk

Rethink Mental Illness

Rethink Mental Illness is a national charity that believes a better life is possible for millions of people affected by mental illness. Their website and helplines give information and advice.

Website: www.rethink.org

The healthtalk webpage on hearing voices

Healthtalkonline is the award-winning website of the DIPEx charity that lets you share in thousands of people's experiences of more than sixty health-related conditions and illnesses. You can watch videos or listen to audio clips of interviews with people who hear voices.

Website: http://www.healthtalkonline.org/mental_health/Experiences_of_psychosis/Topic/3934/

Further reading

Brian Keenan's BBC interview can be downloaded from http://www.bbc.co.uk/sn/tvradio/programmes/horizon/broadband/tx/isolation/keenan/

Overcoming books

Davies, William (2000) *Overcoming Anger & Irritability,* London: Robinson

Fennell, Melanie (1997) *Overcoming Low Self-esteem,* London: Robinson

Freeman, Daniel, Philippa Garety & Jason Freeman (2006) *Overcoming Paranoid & Suspicious Thoughts,* London: Robinson

Gilbert, Paul (2009) *Overcoming Depression* (2nd edn), London: Robinson

Kennerley, Helen (1997) *Overcoming Anxiety,* London: Robinson

Books about voices

Romme, M. & S. Escher (1993) *Accepting Voices,* London: MIND Publications

Romme, M. & S. Escher (2000) *Making Sense of Voices,* London: MIND Publications

Romme, M., S. Escher, J. Dillon, D. Corstens & M. Morris (2009) *Living with Voices: 50 stories of recovery,* Ross-on-Wye: PCCS Books

Books on psychosis

Bentall, R. (2003) *Madness explained: Psychosis and human nature,* London: Penguin Books

Bradstreet, S., R. Chandler & M. Hayward (eds) (2012) *Voicing Carer Experiences,* Scottish Recovery Network

Chandler, R. & M. Hayward (eds) (2009) *Voicing Psychotic Experiences: A reconsideration of recovery and diversity,* Brighton: OLM/Pavilion

Turkington, D., D. Kingdon et al., (2009) *Back to life, back to normality: Cognitive therapy, recovery and psychosis,* Cambridge: Cambridge University Press

Books on assertiveness and mood

Dryden, D. & D. Constantinou (2004) *Assertiveness: Step by Step,* London: Sheldon Press

Greenberger, D. & C.A. Padesky (1995) *Mind over Mood: Change how you feel by changing the way you think,* Guildford Press: London

Appendix

ABC Model referred to section entitled "What do I think about my voice?"

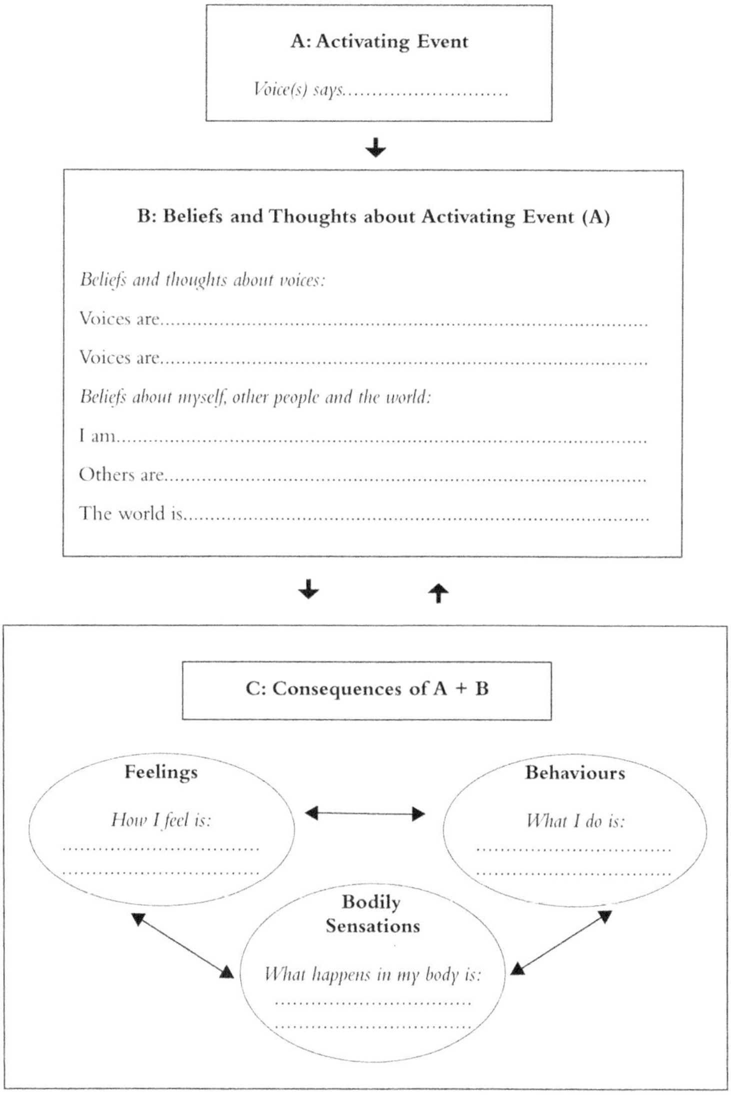

Coping worksheet

- What ways do you use now to cope with your voices?

____

____

____

- How effective are they? Can they make the voices worse? Do they work better at particular times, e.g. when you are – or maybe are not – stressed?

____

____

____

- Do you want to try one or a number of new coping strategies? There are three different types to use (see section entitled "Stress management"):

  * What could you do to manage your stress levels? Try to think of one or two things:

  ____

  ____

  ____

  * Is there anybody you could see? Any social setting? Try to think of one or two:

* Are there any work activities you could try?

* Is there anything that mental health services could offer – such as treatments or other kinds of help – that you might not have tried in the past?

* Sometimes distractions designed to keep your mind occupied can help, e.g. Sudoku, crosswords, music, listening to the radio, computer games. Can you think of one or two you might try?

- Okay – now is the time to select one new coping strategy and decide when you are going to try it, so which one?

- When are you going to do it?

- When you've tried it, check how effective it was:

  * It may not have solved the problem but did it help just a little?

  * Could you have done it differently?

  * Is it worth using it again? Or trying something different?

Rating your self-esteem

[Rosenberg Self-Esteem Scale, Rosenberg 1965]

1. On the whole I am satisfied with myself.

Strongly agree

Agree

Disagree

Strongly Disagree

2. At times, I think I am no good at all.

Strongly agree

Agree

Disagree

Strongly Disagree

3. I feel that I have a number of good qualities.

Strongly agree

Agree

Disagree

Strongly Disagree

---

4. I am able to do things as well as most other people.

Strongly agree

Agree

Disagree

Strongly Disagree

5. I feel I do not have much to be proud of.

Strongly agree

Agree

Disagree

Strongly Disagree

6. I certainly feel useless at times.

Strongly agree

Agree

Disagree

Strongly Disagree

7. I feel that I'm a person of worth, at least on an equal plane with others.

Strongly agree

Agree

Disagree

Strongly Disagree

8. I wish I could have more respect for myself.

Strongly agree

Agree

Disagree

Strongly Disagree

9. All in all, I am inclined to feel that I am a failure.

Strongly agree

Agree

Disagree

Strongly Disagree

10. I take a positive attitude towards myself.

Strongly agree

Agree

Disagree

Strongly Disagree

BAVQ-R

There are many people who hear voices. It would help us to find out how you are feeling about your voices by completing this questionnaire. Please read each statement and tick the box which best describes the way you have been feeling in the *past week.*

If you hear more than one voice, please complete the form for the voice which is dominant.

1

My voice is punishing me for something I have done

Disagree (score 0)

Unsure (score 1)

Slightly Agree (score 2)

Strongly Agree (score 3)

2

My voice wants to help me

Disagree (score 0)

Unsure (score 1)

Slightly Agree (score 2)

Strongly Agree (score 3)

3

My voice is very powerful

Disagree (score 0)

Unsure (score 1)

Slightly Agree (score 2)

Strongly Agree (score 3)

4

My voice is persecuting me for no good reason

Disagree (score 0)

Unsure (score 1)

Slightly Agree (score 2)

Strongly Agree (score 3)

5

My voice wants to protect me

Disagree (score 0)

Unsure (score 1)

Slightly Agree (score 2)

Strongly Agree (score 3)

6

My voice seems to know everything about me

Disagree (score 0)

Unsure (score 1)

Slightly Agree (score 2)

Strongly Agree (score 3)

7

My voice is evil

Disagree (score 0)

Unsure (score 1)

Slightly Agree (score 2)

Strongly Agree (score 3)

8

My voice is helping to keep me sane

Disagree (score 0)

Unsure (score 1)

Slightly Agree (score 2)

Strongly Agree (score 3)

9

My voice makes me do things I really don't want to do

Disagree (score 0)

Unsure (score 1)

Slightly Agree (score 2)

Strongly Agree (score 3)

10

My voice wants to harm me

Disagree (score 0)

Unsure (score 1)

Slightly Agree (score 2)

Strongly Agree (score 3)

11

My voice is helping me to develop my special powers or abilities

Disagree (score 0)

Unsure (score 1)

Slightly Agree (score 2)

Strongly Agree (score 3)

12

I cannot control my voices

Disagree (score 0)

Unsure (score 1)

Slightly Agree (score 2)

Strongly Agree (score 3)

13

My voice wants me to do bad things

Disagree (score 0)

Unsure (score 1)

Slightly Agree (score 2)

Strongly Agree (score 3)

14

My voice is helping me to achieve my goal in life

Disagree (score 0)

Unsure (score 1)

Slightly Agree (score 2)

Strongly Agree (score 3)

15

My voice will harm or kill me if I disobey or resist it

Disagree (score 0)

Unsure (score 1)

Slightly Agree (score 2)

Strongly Agree (score 3)

16

My voice is trying to corrupt or destroy me

Disagree (score 0)

Unsure (score 1)

Slightly Agree (score 2)

Strongly Agree (score 3)

17

I am grateful for my voice

Disagree (score 0)

Unsure (score 1)

Slightly Agree (score 2)

Strongly Agree (score 3)

18

My voice rules my life

Disagree (score 0)

Unsure (score 1)

Slightly Agree (score 2)

Strongly Agree (score 3)

19

My voice reassures me

Disagree (score 0)

Unsure (score 1)

Slightly Agree (score 2)

Strongly Agree (score 3)

20

My voice frightens me

Disagree (score 0)

Unsure (score 1)

Slightly Agree (score 2)

Strongly Agree (score 3)

21

My voice makes me happy

Disagree (score 0)

Unsure (score 1)

Slightly Agree (score 2)

Strongly Agree (score 3)

22

My voice makes me feel down

Disagree (score 0)

Unsure (score 1)

Slightly Agree (score 2)

Strongly Agree (score 3)

23

My voice makes me feel angry

Disagree (score 0)

Unsure (score 1)

Slightly Agree (score 2)

Strongly Agree (score 3)

24

My voice makes me feel calm

Disagree (score 0)

Unsure (score 1)

Slightly Agree (score 2)

Strongly Agree (score 3)

25

My voice makes me feel anxious

Disagree (score 0)

Unsure (score 1)

Slightly Agree (score 2)

Strongly Agree (score 3)

26

My voice makes me feel confident

Disagree (score 0)

Unsure (score 1)

Slightly Agree (score 2)

Strongly Agree (score 3)

When I hear my voice, ***usually***...

27

I tell it to leave me alone

Disagree (score 0)

Unsure (score 1)

Slightly Agree (score 2)

Strongly Agree (score 3)

28

I try and take my mind off it

Disagree (score 0)

Unsure (score 1)

Slightly Agree (score 2)

Strongly Agree (score 3)

29

I try and stop it

Disagree (score 0)

Unsure (score 1)

Slightly Agree (score 2)

Strongly Agree (score 3)

30

I do things to prevent it talking

Disagree (score 0)

Unsure (score 1)

Slightly Agree (score 2)

Strongly Agree (score 3)

31

I listen to it because I want to

Disagree (score 0)

Unsure (score 1)

Slightly Agree (score 2)

Strongly Agree (score 3)

32

I willingly follow what my voice tells me to do

Disagree (score 0)

Unsure (score 1)

Slightly Agree (score 2)

Strongly Agree (score 3)

33

I have done things to start to get in contact with my voice

Disagree (score 0)

Unsure (score 1)

Slightly Agree (score 2)

Strongly Agree (score 3)

34

I seek the advice of my voice

Disagree (score 0)

Unsure (score 1)

Slightly Agree (score 2)

Strongly Agree (score 3)

Malevolence

My voice is punishing me for something I have done
My voice is persecuting me for no good reason
My voice is evil
My voice wants to harm me
My voice wants to do bad things
My voice is trying to corrupt or destroy me

Benevolence

My voice wants to help me
My voice wants to protect me
My voice is helping to keep me sane

My voice is helping me to develop my special powers or abilities
My voice is helping me to achieve my goal in life
I am grateful for my voice

Omnipotence

My voice is very powerful
My voice seems to know everything about me
My voice makes me do things I really don't want to
I cannot control my voices
My voice will kill or harm me if I disobey or resist it
My voice rules my life

Resistance

Feelings

My voice frightens me
My voice makes me feel down
My voice makes me feel angry
My voice makes me feel anxious

Behaviour

I tell it to leave me alone
I try and take my mind of it
I try to stop it

I do things to prevent it talking
I am reluctant to obey it

Engagement

Feelings

My voice reassures me
My voice makes me happy
My voice makes me feel calm
My voice makes me feel anxious

Behaviour

I listen to it because I want to
I willingly follow what my voice tells me to do
I have done things to get in contact with my voice
I seek the advice of my voice

The Voice and You (VAY)

A PERSON'S ASSESSMENT OF THE RELATIONSHIP THEY HAVE WITH THEIR PREDOMINANT VOICE

PLEASE READ THIS BEFORE YOU START

The statements listed here are the sorts of feelings and attitudes which people sometimes have about or towards the voices they hear. Please read each statement carefully and indicate, by ticking the appropriate column, the extent to which you think it applies to you in relation to your predominant voice.

Try to be completely frank and honest about yourself. Avoid answering the way you would like to be or the way you would like others to think of you, rather than the way you really are.

Try as far as possible, to place your ticks in the 'Nearly always true' and 'Rarely true' columns. The two middle columns are really for if you cannot make up your mind.

1. My voice wants things done his/her way

Nearly always true

___

___

___

Quite often true

Sometimes true

Rarely true

2. My voice helps me make up my mind

Nearly always true

Quite often true

Sometimes true

Rarely true

3. I prefer to keep my voice at a safe distance

Nearly always true

Quite often true

Sometimes true

Rarely true

4. My voice makes hurtful remarks to me

Nearly always true

Quite often true

Sometimes true

Rarely true

5. My voice does not let me have time to myself

Nearly always true

Quite often true

Sometimes true

Rarely true

6. I have a tendency to look up to my voice

Nearly always true

Quite often true

Sometimes true

Rarely true

7. When my voice gets too close to me, it makes me feel uneasy

Nearly always true

Quite often true

Sometimes true

Rarely true

8. My voice constantly reminds me of my failings

Nearly always true

Quite often true

Sometimes true

Rarely true

9. My voice dislikes it when I exclude him/her by showing an interest in other people

Nearly always true

Quite often true

Sometimes true

Rarely true

10. I allow my voice to take control of me

Nearly always true

Quite often true

Sometimes true

Rarely true

11. I feel I have little to offer my voice

Nearly always true

Quite often true

Sometimes true

Rarely true

12. It is easy for my voice to change my mind

Nearly always true

Quite often true

Sometimes true

Rarely true

13. My voice does not give me credit for the good things I do

Nearly always true

Quite often true

Sometimes true

Rarely true

14. My voice tries to accompany me when I go out

Nearly always true

Quite often true

Sometimes true

Rarely true

15. I feel deserted when my voice is not around

Nearly always true

Quite often true

Sometimes true

Rarely true

16. I try to hide my feelings from my voice

Nearly always true

Quite often true

Sometimes true

Rarely true

17. My voice tries to get the better of me

Nearly always true

Quite often true

Sometimes true

____
____
____

Rarely true

____
____
____

18. My voice dislikes spending time on his/her own

Nearly always true

____
____
____

Quite often true

____
____
____

Sometimes true

____
____
____

Rarely true

19. My voice's judgment is better than mine

Nearly always true

Quite often true

Sometimes true

Rarely true

20. I do not like to get too involved with my voice

Nearly always true

Quite often true

Sometimes true

Rarely true

21. My voice makes me feel useless

Nearly always true

Quite often true

Sometimes true

Rarely true

22. I need to have my voice around me a great deal

Nearly always true

Quite often true

Sometimes true

Rarely true

23. I don't like my voice to know what I am thinking

Nearly always true

Quite often true

Sometimes true

Rarely true

24. I have difficulty letting go of my voice

Nearly always true

Quite often true

Sometimes true

Rarely true

25. My voice tries to make me out to be stupid

Nearly always true

Quite often true

Sometimes true

______

______

______

Rarely true

______

______

______

26. My voice finds it hard to allow me to have time away from him/her

Nearly always true

______

______

______

Quite often true

______

______

______

Sometimes true

______

______

______

Rarely true

27. I have a great need to talk to my voice

Nearly always true

Quite often true

Sometimes true

Rarely true

28. I don't wish to spend much time listening to my voice

Nearly always true

Quite often true

Sometimes true

Rarely true

Voice And You (VAY)

Items by scale

Voice Dominance

1) My voice wants things done his/her way
4) My voice makes hurtful remarks to me
8) My voice constantly reminds me of my failings
13) My voice does not give me credit for the good things I do
17) My voice tries to get the better of me
21) My voice makes me feel useless
25) My voice tries to make me out to be stupid

Voice Intrusiveness

5) My voice does not let me have time to myself
9) My voice dislikes it when I exclude him/her by showing an interest in other people
14) My voice tries to accompany me when I go out
18) My voice dislikes spending time on his/her own
26) My voice finds it hard to allow me to have time away from him/her

Hearer Dependence

2) My voice helps me make up my mind
6) I have a tendency to look up to my voice
10) I allow my voice to take control of me
12) It is easy for my voice to change my mind
15) I feel deserted when my voice is not around
19) My voice's judgement is better than mine
22) I need to have my voice around me a great deal
24) I have difficulty letting go of my voice
27) I have a great need to talk to my voice

Hearer Distance

3) I prefer to keep my voice at a safe distance
7) When my voice gets too close to me, it makes me feel uneasy
11) I feel I have little to offer my voice
16) I try to hide my feelings from my voice
20) I do not like to get too involved with my voice
23) I don't like my voice to know what I am thinking

28) I don't wish to spend much time listening to my voice

Scoring Guidelines

Scoring

Responses are scored as follows:
Nearly always true=3
Quite often true=2
Sometimes true=1
Rarely true=0

Creating a possible maximum score for each scale of:
Voice dominance=21
Voice intrusiveness=15
Hearer dependence=27
Hearer distance=21

Overcoming Paranoid and Suspicious Thoughts

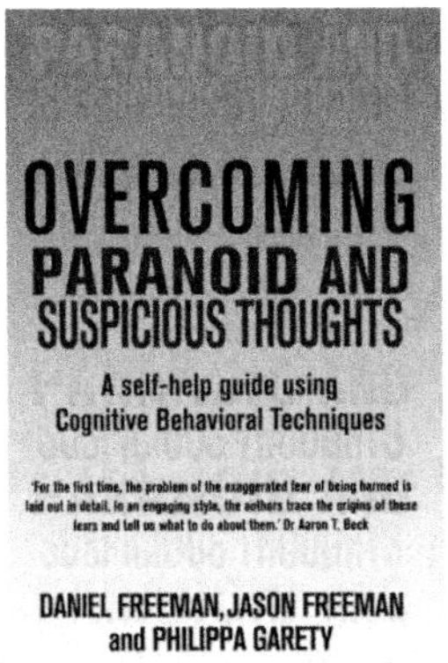

Do you often suspect the worst of others? Mild to moderate paranoia, or mistrust of other people, is on the increase, and although it may feel justifiable at the time, unfounded suspicions of this kind can make life a misery. Research says between 20 and 30 per cent of people in the UK frequently have suspicious or paranoid thoughts. This is the first self-help guide to coping with what can be a debilitating condition.

Visit www.constablerobinson.com for more information

Overcoming Depression

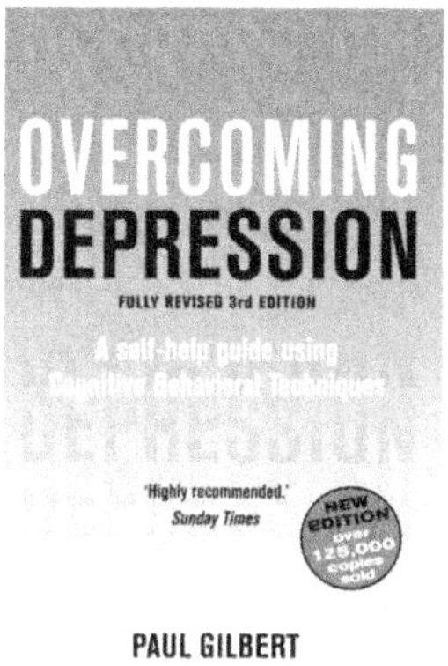

If you suffer from depression you are far from alone. Depression is very common, affecting over 300 million people around the world. Written by Professor Paul Gilbert, internationally recognised for his work on depression, this highly acclaimed self-help book has been of benefit to thousands of people including sufferers, their friends and families, and those working in the medical profession.

This fully revised third edition has been extensively updated and rewritten to reflect over ten years of new research on understanding and treating depression, particularly the importance of developing compassionate ways of thinking, behaving and feeling. It contains helpful case studies and new, easy-to-follow, step-by-step suggestions and exercises to help you understand your depression and lift your mood.

Visit www.constablerobinson.com for more information

Overcoming Low Self-Esteem

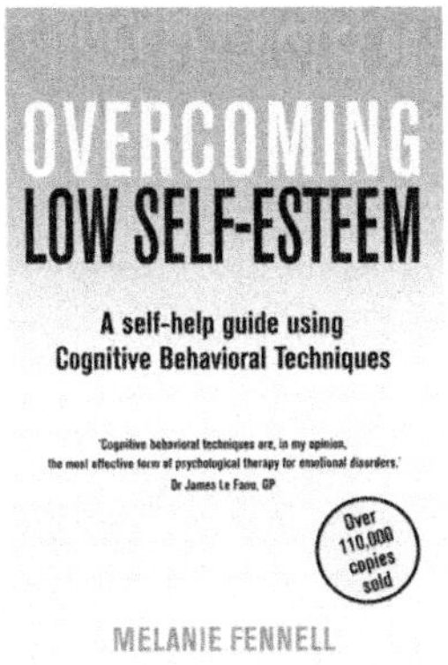

Melanie Fennell's *Overcoming Low Self-Esteem* is a classic of self-help literature, winning acclaim for its practical and user-friendly approach and now recommended on the National Health Service's self-help scheme known as Books on Prescription.

This book will aid readers to understand their condition and with this knowledge enable them to break out of the vicious circle of negative self-image, learn the art of self-acceptance and alter their lives for the better.

Explains the nature of low self-esteem and self-destructive thinking.

Contains a complete self-help programme and monitoring sheets.

Is based on clinically proven techniques of cognitive therapy. Visit www.constablerobinson.com for more information

A

C

W

Printed in Dunstable, United Kingdom

91220102R00212